Focus on Safe Medication Practices

D1374225

Focus on Safe Medication Practices

Melanie J. Rantucci, BScPhm, MScPhm, PhD
Pharmacist Consultant, President
MJR Pharmacy Communications
White Rock, British Columbia
Canada

Christine Stewart, RPh, BScPhm
Pharmacist Consultant, President
Christine Stewart & Associates Inc.
Markham, Ontario
Canada

Ian Stewart, RPh, BScPhm
President
I.R.A.S. Pharmacy Ltd.
Etobicoke, Ontario
Canada

Wolters Kluwer | Lippincott Williams & Wilkins
Health
Philadelphia · Baltimore · New York · London
Buenos Aires · Hong Kong · Sydney · Tokyo

Acquisitions Editor: John Goucher
Managing Editor: Meredith Brittain
Marketing Manager: Christen Murphy
Production Editor: Julie Montalbano
Designer: Stephen Druding
Compositor: Aptara, Inc.

351 West Camden Street   530 Walnut Street
Baltimore, MD 21201   Philadelphia, PA 19106

Printed in China

9 8 7 6 5 4 3   12 11

Library of Congress Cataloging-in-Publication Data

Rantucci, Melanie J.
  Focus on safe medication practices / Melanie J. Rantucci, Christine Stewart, Ian Stewart.
    p. ; cm.
  Includes bibliographical references and index.
  ISBN 978-0-7817-7078-1 (alk. paper)
1. Medication errors—Prevention. I. Stewart, Christine, RPh. II. Stewart, Ian, RPh. III. Title.
  [DNLM: 1. Medication Errors—prevention & control. 2. Pharmaceutical Preparations—adverse effects. 3. Pharmaceutical Services—organization & administration. 4. Risk Management—organization & administration. QV 38 R213f 2009]
  RM146. R36 2009
  615′.6—dc22

                                                              2008011006

DISCLAIMER

Care has been taken to confirm the accuracy of the information present and to describe generally accepted practices. However, the authors, editors, and publisher are not responsible for errors or omissions or for any consequences from application of the information in this book and make no warranty, expressed or implied, with respect to the currency, completeness, or accuracy of the contents of the publication. Application of this information in a particular situation remains the professional responsibility of the practitioner; the clinical treatments described and recommended may not be considered absolute and universal recommendations.

The authors, editors, and publisher have exerted every effort to ensure that drug selection and dosage set forth in this text are in accordance with the current recommendations and practice at the time of publication. However, in view of ongoing research, changes in government regulations, and the constant flow of information relating to drug therapy and drug reactions, the reader is urged to check the package insert for each drug for any change in indications and dosage and for added warnings and precautions. This is particularly important when the recommended agent is a new or infrequently employed drug.

Some drugs and medical devices presented in this publication have Food and Drug Administration (FDA) clearance for limited use in restricted research settings. It is the responsibility of the health care provider to ascertain the FDA status of each drug or device planned for use in their clinical practice.

To purchase additional copies of this book, call our customer service department at **(800) 638-3030** or fax orders to **(301) 223-2320**. International customers should call **(301) 223-2300**.

Visit Lippincott Williams & Wilkins on the Internet: http://www.lww.com. Lippincott Williams & Wilkins customer service representatives are available from 8:30 am to 6:00 pm, EST.

Preface

The primary goal of a health care professional is to provide the best care possible to all patients. In relation to medication, this involves accurately prescribing, dispensing, and administering medications and providing pharmaceutical care. However, because health care professionals are humans working in complex systems, no matter how conscientious, careful, and experienced they are, the potential for a patient to receive an incorrect medication exists. When this occurs, the general response until recently has most often been to focus on *who* is to blame. But who was involved and who is to blame is of far less importance than discovering *what* went wrong, *why,* and *how.* A complete analysis of the what, why, and how enables us to apply the knowledge to similar situations to help prevent future incidents from occurring.

Focus on Safe Medication Practices gives practicing pharmacists, pharmacy technicians, and pharmacy students, as well as other health professionals, an overview of the risks of various types of medication incidents and preventive strategies. It should be used as an adjunct to comprehensive training in communication skills and dispensing procedures to optimally improve patient safety. While written primarily for the North American health care and medication use system, the issues discussed in this book apply to most countries to varying degrees. For pharmacy and pharmacy technician students, this book will provide an overview as well as specific examples of medication incidents and preventive strategies.

Medication incidents can happen in all types of practices, but some errors relate to specific environments. For example, hospital pharmacies have a much higher use of intravenous drugs than community pharmacies, so there is greater chance of incidents involving calculations of IV dosages and incorrect administration sites. The data in the literature relates primarily to the hospital environment because most hospitals have policies that require reporting of medication incidents. But the literature dealing with causes of incidents applies to both community and hospital environments. The information contained in this resource is applicable to pharmacists and pharmacy technicians wherever they practice as well as to other health professionals involved in the medication use system.

GOALS OF THIS BOOK

The overall goal of this book is to examine why medication errors happen and how they can be prevented in the future, with the ultimate aim of improving patient safety in relation to medication use. In order to do that, this book is structured around the eight objectives discussed below.

Objective 1: To Be Aware of the Issue

Patient safety in relation to medication use is an issue that hits close to home for health professionals and is a theme throughout this book. Few pharmacists and technicians can say they have never been involved in a medication error, even if that error did not result in harm. They generally feel uncomfortable with the topic of medication incidents. There is a lot of emotion attached to the subject, including guilt, fear, anger, shame, and the desire to blame or punish someone for the error.

However reluctant they may feel, health professionals need to be aware of the issues and to become comfortable with learning about and discussing medication incidents. They also need to be aware of the need to identify the risk of medication incidents and to accept responsibility for their role in actions to prevent and manage medication incidents.

Objective 2: To Become Familiar with the Terminology

In order to discuss the issues involved in medication incidents, readers need to be familiar with various terms relating to such events. In reading studies and various articles relating to the issue, one can become confused if terms are not clearly defined, and comparisons of statistics become impossible. Therefore definitions of major terms are presented in Chapter 1, and a glossary appears at the end of this book. The authors have made every effort to be consistent throughout the book in the use of these terms.

Objective 3: To Understand the Scope and Frequency of Medication Incidents

To better understand the scope of the issue, it is helpful to review the current state of affairs. Reports in the United States, Britain, Australia and Canada have pointed out that a wide range of adverse events can and do occur when patients enter the health care system, resulting in great personal and financial costs to patients and the system. A large percentage of these adverse events, many of which are preventable, result from medication usage. Subsequently, studies have been conducted in various countries to assess the frequency of medical errors and medication incidents in hospitals and community pharmacies. To a lesser degree, the causes of these incidents have been explored. Chapter 1 provides a review of these reports and studies to provide perspective and raise awareness of the need for knowledge and actions by health professionals, as discussed in subsequent chapters.

Objective 4: To Identify Common Types of Errors Relating to Medication

Because the medication provision and use system is complex, there are ample opportunities for mistakes to be made. Experts have developed theories to help explain why errors occur and to identify contributory factors, and these theories have been applied to the medication use system.

To systematize the problems relating to medication errors, analysts have identified the steps, procedures, and people who may be involved. In addition, they have classified the types of errors so that causes can be pinpointed and steps to prevention can be identified and acted upon. Chapter 2 describes the theory of error and various contributory factors and the classification of types of errors. Chapters 4, 5, and 6 discuss specific examples of errors.

Objective 5: To Recognize Medication Incidents Specific to Certain Specialty Areas

Some types of patients, medications, and environments present particular risks in regard to medication incidents. Health professionals in specialty practices (for example, pediatrics) need to be aware of issues that raise risks in these types of practices. Chapter 6 discusses potential errors and preventative measures for specialty areas.

Objective 6: To Implement Measures to Reduce the Risk of Medication Incidents

Health professionals, pharmaceutical manufacturers, governments, institutions, and patients all have a role in reducing medications incidents. An overview of risk analysis and numerous preventive strategies appear in Chapter 3. Next, Chapters 4, 5, and 6 discuss preventive strategies for specific types of errors. Chapter 7 discusses preventive strategies involving the use of technology, and Chapter 9, in addition to summarizing many of these measures, discusses the implementation of safe medication practices in the pharmacy.

Objective 7: To Identify Potential Sources of Error

To better understand and prevent errors, it is helpful to examine specific examples and situations. Chapters 4 and 5 discuss in detail the potential causes of specific types of errors and strategies for their prevention. Chapter 6 includes examples of errors specific to various specialty areas. Chapter 7 describes potential errors related to technology used in the medication system.

Objective 8: Dealing with a Medication Incident

With the identification and analysis of risk and the implementation of various preventive strategies, medication incidents will decrease. How each incident is handled is crucial to the outcome of the incident and to the prevention of future incidents. Chapter 8 presents a procedure for handling incidents, communication strategies following an incident, and analysis of the incident.

PEDAGOGICAL FEATURES

To assist readers in learning, the following features are included in this book:

- **Objectives:** Each chapter starts with a list of objectives and proceeds logically to accomplish them.
- **Case studies:** Where appropriate, case studies have been inserted to illustrate the material being discussed. There are many descriptions of specific medication incidents, including a description of the incident, contributing factors, and preventive strategies. The book also contains situations describing interactions involving pharmacists and patients to illustrate the human and communication aspects of medication incidents.
- **Reflective questions:** These appear at the end of each chapter to allow readers to reflect on the material in the chapter in relation to particular patients and situations, or in terms of their own practices.

Reviewers

Cheryl Aiken, BS, PharmD, RPh
Hotel Pharmacy
Brattleboro, Vermont

Bernadette K. Brown, BS, PharmD
Butler University College of
  Pharmacy and Health Sciences
Indianapolis, Indiana

Sherrill Brown, DVM, PharmD
Director, Drug Information Service
Assistant Professor, Pharmacy
  Practice
University of Montana
Missoula, Montana

**George W. Fakhoury, MD, DORCP,
  CMA (AAMA)**
Curriculum Manger
Heald College, LLC
San Francisco, California

Jan K. Hastings, PharmD
Pharmacy Practice Department
University of Arkansas for Medical
  Sciences
College of Pharmacy
Little Rock, Arkansas

Susan Jay, RPh
Associate Professor
Pharmacy Practice and Science
  Department
University of Kentucky
Lexington, Kentucky

Shawna Lopez, CPhT
BAAS in Biology
Director Pharmacy Technology
Amarillo College
Amarillo, Texas

Jeanetta Mastron, BS, CPhT
Pharmacy Technician Program
  Educator/Director
American University of Health
  Sciences
Long Beach, California

Nancy L. Needham, CPhT
Associate of Science in Pharmacy
  Technology
Bachelor of Science in Health
  Science
Master of Arts in Education
American Career College
Anaheim, California

**Joanne O'Connell Whitney, PhD,
  PharmD**
University of California,
  San Francisco
San Francisco, California

Mark Williams, BS
Coordinator
Pharmacy Technology Department
Mercy College of Northwest Ohio
Toledo, Ohio

Acknowledgments

We would like to thank Wayne Caverly of WMC Efficient Pharmacy Solutions Inc., 2604 Royal Mews, Ste. Lazare, Quebec, for writing Chapter 7 "Technology Solutions to Promote Safe Medication Practices," which we asked him to contribute to the book because of his breadth of knowledge and experience in this field. Thanks also to the reviewers and in particular to Cheryl Aiken for reviewing the content to ensure that it is appropriate for U.S. pharmacists.

We would also like to acknowledge *Pharmacy Practice* (a Rogers Media publication) and McKesson Canada for supporting an earlier version of this book, a booklet entitled *Safe Medication Practices: A Pharmacist's Guide to Preventing and Managing Medication Incidents*, printed in Canada in 2004 and distributed to pharmacies in Canada by McKesson Canada.

Acknowledgment

Contents

Chapter 5: Underlying Root Causes and Preventive Strategies   74

Chapter 6: Causes and Preventive Strategies in Specialty Practices 105

Chapter 7: Technological Solutions Promoting Safe
Medication Practices   123

Chapter 8: Dealing with Medication Incidents in Pharmacy   149

Chapter 9: Instituting Safe Medication Practices in Pharmacy   177

Appendix A: Organizations Involved in Patient Safety   197

Appendix B: Strategies and Tools for Prevention of Specific Types of Problems   200

Chapter 1

Defining the Issues

Objectives

After completing this chapter, the reader will be able to:

- Explain the need for health professionals to identify the risk, accept the responsibility, and take action to prevent and manage medication incidents
- Define terms used in discussions of medication incidents
- Refer to international reports recognizing the issue of medical error
- Refer to studies identifying medical and medication errors
- Describe the impact of medication errors

In the past, the subject of **medication errors** was strictly taboo—health care professionals did not discuss the issue in open forums, even though they knew it was a problem. As a result, many of the same types of **errors** have occurred repeatedly because of a lack of awareness of those errors and because nothing was being done to prevent them from being repeated. More recently, a greater awareness and openness regarding **patient safety** and all types of **medical errors** has arisen among health professionals and the public alike, to the point where even the popular media have taken up the issue. An excerpt from the popular magazine *Time* in December 1999, titled "Doctors' Deadly Mistakes," asserts: "Depending on which statistics you believe, the number of Americans killed by medical screw-ups is somewhere between 44,000 and 98,000 every year—the eighth leading cause of death even by the more conservative figure, ahead of car crashes, breast cancer and AIDS."[1]

Health care organizations and health professionals have come to realize that other industries and sectors of the economy have made efforts to identify high risks and made progress in error reduction and safety assurance.[2] The aviation, nuclear, and military communities along with manufacturing sectors and such companies as Motorola and General Electric have studied and monitored error and taken action to reduce and prevent it.[2]

In light of such increased awareness of errors, health professionals have begun to take notice. Various groups and organizations involved in health care have been studying the frequency and causes of errors. They have suggested potential preventive strategies and made recommendations to improve patient safety. Medication errors are the most common medical errors, injuring millions of people and costing billions of dollars annually.[3] Pharmacists, pharmacy technicians, and other health professionals who are responsible for providing and managing medications are key in preventing **adverse events** involving medications. To do this, they need to be aware of the issues involved in medication

1

safety, the many factors causing **medication incidents,** the types of errors that can occur, and preventive strategies.

DEFINITIONS

In order to fully understand the issue of medication incidents, one must first be familiar with the terms and definitions used. This can be confusing, since there are many different terms and definitions. The World Health Organization (WHO) has noted that it is imperative to develop common definitions.[4]

In the broader area of the health care system, the term **patient safety** is defined as the "freedom from accidental injuries during the course of medical care; activities to avoid, prevent or correct adverse outcomes which may result from delivery of health care."[5] An **adverse event** covers everything that can go wrong with a patient in the health care system, not just medication-related events. It is defined as an injury that is the unintended result of medical management and includes all kinds of adverse outcomes associated with medical care, such as **iatrogenic** illnesses, therapeutic problems, and untoward incidents.[5,6]

In terms of problems specific to the use of medications, an **adverse drug event** is an injury occurring during the patient's drug therapy and resulting either from appropriate care or from unsuitable or suboptimal care. It includes both adverse drug reactions during normal use of the medicine and any harm resulting from a medication error, both **errors of omission and of commission.**"[5] Thus a **medication error** is one of several causes of an adverse drug event and is defined as an error involving inappropriate medication use or patient harm as a result of a preventable problem in the medication use process.[7-9] It can be an error in prescribing, order communication, product labeling, packaging, nomenclature, compounding, dispensing, distribution, administration, education, monitoring, and use. It can occur while the medication is in the control of a health care professional, patient, or caregiver.

There are other terms used for errors, such as **mistake, lapse,** and **slip**, and terms such as **drug misadventure, dispensing error, preparation error, administration error,** and **prescribing error,** which further describe the circumstances.[5,10] Other terms, such as **near miss, close call,** or **medication discrepancy,** refer to situations where the error was detected before it affected the patient.[2,6]

The appropriate use of terms is important to openly discuss and address the issues involved in patient safety. The word "error," in particular, has negative connotations and is associated with blaming individuals rather than the various causes that may be responsible within the system. Terms such as **incident** and **sentinel event** are increasingly being used in place of "error" because it is felt that they better serve to support an environment that encourages reporting, learning, and change. It has also been recommended that we avoid terms such as "accident, "blame," "fault," **negligence,** and "recklessness" in discussing patient safety because they seek to assign blame rather than improve a system (although the last two terms are often used in legal and professional regulatory proceedings).[11] A glossary of terms is included at the end of this book.

TYPES OF MEDICATION INCIDENTS

The description of what constitutes an actual incident can also be confusing. In any program reporting or preventing incidents, it is critical to clarify this for everyone participating. The National Coordinating Council has developed a Taxonomy of Medication Errors for Medication Errors Reporting and Prevention (NCC-MERP).[12] The U.S. Food and Drug Administration (FDA) MedWatch program has adopted this for documenting all cases of medication errors reported. It includes 16 types of "errors" as well as a category titled "other." These are shown in Table 1.1 with asterisks after them.[12]

The NCC-MERP list covers medication incidents involving the dispensing and administration of a medication. However, given the glossary of terms discussed above and in order to allow for near misses, one might also include transcribing errors, product **labeling errors,** and **prescribing errors** as well as a multitude of less visible errors.[13] Most studies focus on medication safety issues constituting **errors of commission** that occur as a result of actions such as dispensing, since they are most visible. However, ideally, issues of medication effectiveness or access to drug therapy that constitute **errors of omission** should also be addressed.[14] Examples of this are failure to adjust the dose in response to a laboratory test value or lack of anticoagulation therapy in immobilized patients to prevent thrombosis.[14] Thus a more complete list of medication incident types might also include these categories (see Table 1.1).

STUDIES OF PATIENT SAFETY

Having defined the terms, we can begin to define the problem. Concern for patient safety was documented as early as the 17th century B.C. in the Code of Hammurabi and later by Hippocrates.[15] Studies reporting adverse events can be found a century ago in the *Journal of the American Medical Association,* with studies increasing throughout the 1950s and 1960s. There continued to be little interest in the United States until a larger body of evidence emerged in 1991, when the results of the Harvard Medical Practice Study were published.[4] Australia, Great Britain, and the United States also embarked on studies and reports that brought the issue of patient safety to the forefront of debate throughout the world.[4] Canada, Denmark, the Netherlands, Sweden, and New Zealand also followed suit.[4,15] By 2003, almost 1% of the National Library of Medicine's electronic database (PubMed) involved publications dealing with patient safety or medical errors.[15]

There are several levels of investigation into the issue of patient safety: reports on the broad issue of patient safety; studies of adverse medical events, which include all incidents (not just medications) adversely affecting a patient in the health care system; and studies of medication errors in hospitals and community pharmacies.

TABLE 1.1
Types of Medication Incidents

- Omission of dose*
- Extra dose*
- Noncompliance*
- Over or under dosage*
- Incorrect dose*
- Incorrect strength/concentration*
- Incorrect drug*
- Incorrect dosage form*
- Incorrect technique*
- Incorrect administration route*
- Incorrect duration*
- Incorrect dosing time*
- Incorrect rate of administration*
- Incorrect patient*
- Error in monitoring*
- Deteriorated drug*
- Drug–drug interaction
- Drug–disease interaction
- Error in transcribing
- Incorrect labeling of product
- Incorrect labeling of dispensed drug
- Error in prescribing
- Drug prescribed for known allergy
- Lack of preventive therapy
- Failure to adjust drug dose as needed

*Included in *Taxonomy of Medication Errors* developed by NCC-MERP.
Sources: Thomas M, Holquist C, Phillips J. Med error reports to FDA show a mixed bag. FDA Safety Page. *Drug Topics.* 2001;1:23. Available at www.fda.gov/cder/drug/MedErrors/mixed.pdf (accessed June 2006); Hicks R, Cousins D, Williams R. Selected medication-error data from USP's MEDMARX program for 2002. *Am J Health Syst Pharm.* 2004;61(10):993–1000.

Reports on Patient Safety

Government-sponsored reports on the safety of patients while under medical care have been published in a number of countries in recent years, including the United States, Canada, Australia, and the United Kingdom.[4,11,15] The 1999 U.S. Institute of Medicine (IOM) report *To Err is Human, Building a Safer*

Health System—Focusing on the Quality of Health Care in America, discusses medical errors occurring in hospitals (excluding clinics, pharmacies, doctors' offices, nursing homes, and outpatient centers). It documents the number of medical errors affecting patient care, the root causes of medical error, the parties responsible for error, and ways to make the system safer.[16] The IOM report estimates that 44,000 to 100,000 Americans die in hospitals annually from adverse events. It calls for a 50% reduction in medical errors over the following 5 years and advocates a move away from the "shame and blame" approach.

The 1999 IOM report was followed up in 2006 with another report entitled *Preventing Medication Errors,* focusing on medications.[17] It found that medication errors are "surprisingly common and costly" and set forth "a comprehensive approach to decreasing the prevalence of these errors," including required changes from doctors, nurses, pharmacists, and others in the health care industry, the FDA, other government agencies, hospitals, other health care organizations, and patients.[18] Recommendations from this report are discussed further in Chapter 3.

The World Health Organization (WHO) addressed the issue of patient safety internationally in its 2002 *Report on Quality of Care: Patient Safety*.[4] It noted that adverse events are "a significant avoidable cause of human suffering that take a high toll in financial loss and opportunity cost to health services."[4] The report called for health systems to promote patient safety; develop standards and guidelines; support reporting systems, preventive action, and measures to reduce risk; and promote evidence-based policies and a **culture of safety.**[4]

Studies of Adverse Medical Events

Surveys of the public and hospital chart reviews have further revealed adverse medical events. A summary of some recent studies in the United States and internationally is shown in Table 1.2. Although populations and health care systems differ somewhat between countries, the results were surprisingly similar, showing that this is an international issue shared by all countries. A survey conducted in 2002 by the Commonwealth Fund in Australia, Canada, New Zealand, the United Kingdom, and the United States asked sicker adults about medical and medication errors experienced in the preceding 2 years.[19] Those reporting that they believed a medical mistake had been made in their treatment or care ranged from 13% (United Kingdom) to 23% (United States).[19]

Studies of patients' hospital charts reveal rates of medical adverse events from 2.9% (United States) to 16.6% (Australia); of those events, from 37% (Canada and New Zealand) to 51% (Australia) are deemed preventable.[15]

The *Harvard Medical Practice Study found that 3.7% of patients experienced* an adverse event and 13.6% of those injuries were fatal. Sixty-nine percent of the injuries were due to errors (i.e., preventable).[20] Further analysis revealed that drugs accounted for 19.4% of the adverse events.

Studies of ambulatory patients are rare, but a 2004 Canadian study of patients discharged from hospital during a 14-week interval found that 23%

TABLE 1.2
Studies of Adverse Medical Events

Authors/Date	Design	Results
Commonwealth Fund, 2002.[19]	Survey of sicker adults over 18 with serious illness or injury and treatment in the past 2 years in hospital	13% (UK) to 23% (U.S.) reported a medical mistake had happened to them. 10% (UK) to 13% (New Zealand) received a wrong medication or wrong dose. 51% (UK) to 63% (U.S.) of those reporting a medical mistake believed that it had caused a serious health problem.
Brennan et al., 1984.[20]	Population-based study from chart reviews in 51 hospitals in New York State	3.7% of patients experienced an adverse event resulting in an injury that prolonged stay or caused disability. 13.6% of those injuries were fatal. 69% of the injuries were due to errors (i.e., preventable). 31% were considered unavoidable. Drugs accounted for 19.4% of the adverse events. Other classes of adverse events were diagnostic (8.1%), therapeutic (7.5%), procedure-related (7%), surgical (47.7%) and other (10.3%).
Forster et al., 2004.[21]	Study of patients discharged from the general internal medicine service during a 14-week interval	23% experienced an adverse event after discharge. 72% of those adverse events were medication-related.

experienced an adverse event after discharge.[21] Seventy-two percent of those adverse events were medication-related.[21]

Studies of Adverse Drug Events

Studies of medication-related adverse events have been conducted in hospital and community pharmacies. A summary of some recent studies is shown in Table 1.3.

The reporting in hospital studies generally comprises all types of adverse events, including unpreventable (adverse effects) and preventable (medication errors) ones. A 1995 U.S. study reviewed hospital admissions, finding that 6.5% of admitted patients experienced an adverse drug event.[22] In an analysis of **preventable adverse drug events (pADEs),** 28% were found to be due to

TABLE 1.3

Studies of Adverse Drug Events from Hospitals and Community Pharmacies

Authors/Date	Design	Results
Bates et al., 1995.[22]	U.S. study reviewed 4,032 hospital admissions	6.5% of patients experienced an ADE.* 5.5% potential adverse drug events. 1% of those fatal, 12% life-threatening, 30% serious. 42% of life-threatening and serious adverse drug events were preventable.
Leape et al., 1995.[23]	Analysis of above study results of preventable adverse drug events (pADE),	28% ADEs due to errors (pADE).† 21% in more than 1 stage of the drug use process. Most in prescribing (39%) and administration (38%).
Kanjanarat et al., 2003.[14]	Review of international studies published between 1994 and 2001 analyzing adverse drug events in hospitals in various countries involving over 117,000 patients	Median 1.8% preventable adverse drug events (pADEs) (1.3–7.8 events per 100 patients). 56% during prescribing; 34% administering; 6% transcribing; 4% dispensing. Most common types of pADEs: 22.4% dosing; 17% inappropriate drug or wrong choice of drugs; 16.5% inappropriate drug administration; 12% inadequate or lack of patient monitoring; 8.8% wrong frequency or wrong time.
Johnston et al., 1993.[25]	Dispensing errors in U.S. Veterans Administration medical centers	21.7 incidents per 100,000 units dispensed.
Flynn et al., 2003.[26]	Observational study of community pharmacies, in 50 pharmacies in 6 U.S. cities studied dispensing errors on new and refill prescriptions.	87.2% to 100% accuracy rates, average 98.3%. 77 errors in 4,481 prescriptions: 5 (6.5%) clinically important. Most common: wrong label information and instructions.
Quinlan et al., 2002.[27]	Study of potential errors intercepted by pharmacists in 34 British pharmacies	0.69% intervention rate: 9.5% dosing (15% potentially serious); 8.1% drug strength (10.9% potentially serious); 3.1% potential adverse reactions (21.8% potentially serious); 2.2% potential drug interactions (10.9% potentially serious).
Santell et al., 2005.[28]	USP MEDMARX voluntary, self-reports by pharmacists	235,159 reports of errors detected for the year 2003.

*ADE, adverse drug event.
†pADE, preventable adverse drug event.

errors.[23] Most of those errors occurred in the prescribing and administration stage.[23]

A review of international studies analyzing adverse drug events in hospitals found a median frequency of 1.8% preventable adverse drug events (pADEs).[14] Most pADEs occurred in the prescribing stage of the drug use process. The most common types of pADEs reported were dosing errors, which included missed doses and wrong or inappropriate doses.[14]

Despite differences in the setting, assessment criteria, and definitions, the nature and percentages of pADEs are quite similar; however, they depend on health care professionals' ability to recognize errors.[14] Because of the nature of the reporting, there is also a bias toward errors of commission, such as adverse drug reactions (ADRs) or overdoses, whereas errors of omission, such as access to drug therapy and effectiveness, were rarely addressed.

Other studies have calculated error rates during medication dispensing. Depending on how they are measured, how they are gathered (e.g., anonymously, chart review, observation, self-report, incident reports) and what is included (e.g., whether they include missed doses, near misses, wrong time, etc.), error rates vary.[24] Thus one can find estimates of one error per patient per day; 0.04% to 2.9% of doses dispensed during the medication cart-filling process; or 1.5% to 4% of prescriptions filled for ambulatory patients.[24]

A study of hospital dispensing errors in U.S. Veterans Administration medical centers revealed 21.7 incidents per 100,000 units dispensed.[25] Studies of outpatient pharmacies have detected error rates ranging from 0.2% to 10% of prescriptions dispensed.[26] A study of 50 U.S. community pharmacies found accuracy rates ranging from 87.2% to 100%, with an average of 98.3%.[26] This translates to an estimated 51.5 million errors (3.3 million potentially important) in 3 billion prescriptions dispensed in the United States per year.[26]

Thankfully, many errors are detected before they affect the patient. A study of potential errors resulting from prescriptions and intercepted by pharmacists in 34 British pharmacies found a 0.69% intervention rate.[27]

Pharmacists are aware of actual and potential errors that occur in practice and share them with other pharmacists through databases of medication errors such as the U.S. Pharmacopeia's MEDMARX, the FDA's Adverse Event Reporting System (AERS), and the National Coordinating Council for Medication Errors Reporting and Prevention (NCC-MERP). These present a slightly different picture, as they are voluntary, self-reports of detected errors. USP MEDMARX had 235,159 reports of errors in 2003.[28]

THE IMPACT OF ADVERSE DRUG EVENTS AND MEDICATION ERRORS

Table 1.4 illustrates the impact of adverse drug events and medications errors in the United States by the numbers. Both the public and health professionals were shocked when the U.S. IOM report estimated that 44,000 to 100,000 Americans die in hospitals annually from adverse events and 7,000 die per year

TABLE 1.4
The Numbers Show the Impact of Adverse Events

44,000 to 100,000	Number of Americans who die in hospitals per year from adverse events[16]
7,000	Number of Americans who die per year from medication usage[16]
$17 billion to $29 billion (USD)	Estimated cost per year of all preventable adverse medical events including lost income, disability and medical expenses[16]
1.5	Percent of reported adverse drug events that resulted in some level of harm (reported to USP MEDMARX in 2003)[28]
129	Number of serious medication errors out of 273 reports to FDA AERS in a month; 18 fatal; 12 life-threatening; 8 associated with disability, 56 required hospitalization, and 35 required intervention to prevent permanent impairment[13]
34.4	Allergic or skin reactions as a percent of preventable adverse drug events (pADE) in hospitals[14]
14.3	Hepatotoxicity or nephrotoxicity as a percent of pADE in hospitals[14]
13.2	Cardiovascular system effects as a percent of pADE in hospitals[14]
13.2	Hematological effects as a percent of pADE in hospitals[13]
10.5	Central nervous system effects as a percent of pADE in hospitals[14]

because of improper medication usage.[16] The financial costs of all preventable adverse medical events in the United States, including lost income, disability, and medical expenses, was estimated in 1999 to be between $17 billion and $29 billion (USD).[16]

The impact in terms of harm to individuals from reported adverse events varies in severity. Only 1.5% of adverse drug events reported to USP MEDMARX in 2003 resulted in some level of harm.[28] However, harm can range from fatal to life-threatening or disabling, requiring hospitalization or requiring intervention to prevent permanent impairment.[13]

Preventable adverse drug events (pADEs) in hospitals most frequently result in allergic or skin reactions, followed by hepatotoxicity or nephrotoxicity, effects on the cardiovascular system (e.g., bradycardia or hypotension), hematological effects (e.g., bleeding or electrolyte imbalances), and central nervous system effects (e.g., confusion or oversedation).[14]

However, percentages and statistics do not tell the whole story of the impact of adverse drug events. The disastrous effects on individual patients make the most compelling case for pharmacists to take action to prevent medication incidents. A number of notable cases highlight the personal tragedy that can result from adverse drug events.

In 2006, three babies died and three were in critical condition after receiving overdoses of heparin at Methodist Hospital in Indianapolis, Indiana.[29] This occurred when adult doses of heparin were accidentally stored in the neonatal unit's drug cabinet. Tragically, this was not the first time heparin overdoses had occurred; the previous two cases had fortunately recovered. In the same hospital in the same year, an 18-year-old received 122 mL of painkiller in an epidural administered over 1 hour instead of 10 hours due to an improperly programmed pump.[30] As a result, the patient temporarily lost feeling and movement in her legs.

In 2001, the *Washington Post* reported the tragic death of a 9-month-old baby girl because of a decimal point error in which prescribed morphine ".5 mg" IV was transcribed to "5 mg,"—another frequently reported error.[31]

In 1997, an 80-year-old grandmother was undergoing tests at Community Hospital in Santa Rosa, California, when undiluted potassium chloride instead of saline solution was used to clean the intravenous line leading to her heart, resulting in death within seconds.[32] Three months later, another 80-year-old woman died at Santa Rosa Memorial Hospital after being accidentally injected with undiluted potassium chloride.[32] These deaths occurred even though the hazards of concentrated potassium chloride were well known and reported on widely, including warnings from the Institute for Safe Medication Practices and numerous journal articles.

These cases put a human face on the tragedy of medication incidents and force health professionals to face up to these problems as well as resolve to take action to ensure safe medication practices. They also illustrate that similar incidents occur repeatedly in spite of reporting and awareness among health professionals. Clearly, we need to understand more about what causes medication errors and what actions can effectively prevent them.

SUMMARY

Reviewing the current information from the United States and around the world, as detailed above, one can see that we know relatively little that can help us to prevent medication incidents. We do not know what strategies are most effective in reducing the rate and impact of specific types of adverse events in different care settings and communities. In addition, we do not know if effective strategies are being implemented. Research is ongoing regarding effective strategies to improve patient safety, but until then pharmacists and pharmacy technicians must learn all they can from existing data. We should not use the numbers and percentages reported here to compare practice sites or pharmacist quality, since **there are no acceptable incidence rates for medication errors.** Rather, we should learn as much as possible from them and develop strategies to prevent them.[8]

The following chapters will provide some strategies that we can put in place to help reduce medication incidents and improve medication safety.

Reflective Questions

1. What is the effect of using terms such as "error" and "fault" in discussing medication incidents?
2. Discuss three reasons why pharmacists should learn about medication incidents.
3. Describe the different types of studies and statistics that define patient safety issues.

REFERENCES

1. Lemonick MD. Doctors' deadly mistakes. *Time.* December 13, 1999. Available at: www.time.com/magazine/article/0,9171,992809,00.html. Accessed January 24, 2008.
2. Quality Interagency Coordination Task Force. Doing What Counts for Patient Safety: Federal Actions to Reduce Medical Errors and Their Impact. Report of the Quality Interagency Coordination Task Force to the President, February 2000 (QuIC). Available at: www.quic.gov/Report/toc.htm. Accessed January 24, 2008.
3. National Academies. Medication errors injure 1.5 million people and cost billions of dollars annually. *News.* July 20, 2006. Available at: www8.nationalacademies.org/onpinews/newsitem.aspx?RecordID=11623. Accessed January 24, 2008.
4. Secretariat of the World Health Organization. Quality of Care: Patient Safety; Report to the 55th World Health Assembly. Geneva: WHO, 2002.
5. Committee of Experts on Management of Safety and Quality in Health Care Expert Group on Safe Medication Practices, Council of Europe. Glossary of Terms Related to Patient and Medication Safety. Geneva: WHO;, 2005. Available at: www.who.int/patientsafety/highlights/COE_patient_and_medication_safety_gl.pdf. Accessed July 6, 2006.
6. United States Department of Veteran's Affairs. National Center for Patient Safety. Glossary of Patient Safety Terms. Available at: www.va.gov/ncps/glossary.html. Accessed January 24, 2008.
7. National Coordinating Council for Medication Error and Prevention: NCCMERP. Available at: www.nccmerp.org. Accessed January 24, 2008
8. Institute for Safe Medication Practices (ISMP). Frequently Asked Questions. Available at: www.ismp.org/faq.asp. Accessed January 24, 2008.
9. U.S. Food and Drug Administration. Center for Drug Evaluation and Research. Medication Errors. Available at: www.fda.gov/cder/drug/MedErrors/default.htm Accessed January 24, 2008.
10. Reason JT. *Human Error.* New York: Cambridge University Press; 1990:9.
11. Royal College of Physicians and Surgeons of Canada. Building a Safer System—A National Integrated Strategy for Improving Patient Safety in Canadian Health Care. National Steering Committee on Patient Safety, Sept 2002. Available at: http://books.nap.edu/openbook.php?isbn=0309068371. Accessed February 2008.
12. Hicks R, Cousins D, Williams R. Selected medication-error data from USP's MEDMARX program for 2002. *Am J Health Syst Pharm.* 2004;61(10):993–1000.
13. Thomas M, Holquist C, Phillips J. Med error reports to FDA show a mixed bag. FDA Safety Page. *Drug Topics.* 2001;1:23. Available at: www.fda.gov/cder/drug/MedErrors/mixed.pdf. Accessed June 2006.
14. Kanjanarat P, Winterstein A, Johns T, et al. Nature of preventable adverse drug events in hospitals: a literature review. *Am J Health Syst Pharm.* 2003;60(14):1750–1759.

15. Canadian Institute for Health Information. Patient safety—a worldwide challenge. In: Health Care in Canada 2004. Canadian Institute for Health Information; 2004: 29–38. Available at: http://secure.cihi.ca/cihiweb/products/hcic2004_chap3_e.pdf. Accessed July 11, 2006.

16. Kohn LT, Corrigan JM, et al., eds. *To Err is Human: Building a Safer Health System.* Washington, DC: National Academy Press, Institute of Medicine; 1999. Available at: www.nap.edu/html/to_err_ is_ human. Accessed May 2, 2004.

17. Institute of Medicine. National Academy of Sciences. *Preventing Medication Errors.* Washington, DC: National Academies Press; 2006. Available at: www.nap.edu/ CMS/3809/22526/35939.aspx. Accessed September 2006.

18. Institute of Medicine. Preventing Medication Errors. Report Brief. July 2006. Available at: www.iom.edu/Object.File/Master/35/943/medications%20errors%20new.pdf/. Accessed September 2006.

19. Blendon RJ, Schoen C, DesRoches C, et al. Common concerns amid diverse systems: health care experiences in five countries. *Health Affairs.* 2003;22(3):106–121.

20. Brennan T, Leape LL, Laird N, et al. Nature of adverse events in hospitalized patients. Results of the Harvard Medical Practice Study II. *N Engl J Med.* 1991;324(6):377–384.

21. Forster A, Clark H, Menard A, et al. Adverse events among medical patients after discharge from hospital. *CMAJ.* 2004;170(3):345–349.

22. Bates DW, Cullen D, Laird N, et al. Incidence of adverse drug events and potential adverse drug events. Implication for prevention. *JAMA.* 1995;274(1):29–34.

23. Leape LL, Bates DW, Cullen DJ, et al. Systems analysis of adverse drug events. *JAMA.* 1995;274(1):35–43.

24. Flynn E, Barker K. Medication errors research. In: Cohen M, ed. *Medication Errors: Causes, Prevention and Risk Management.* Boston: Jones and Bartlett; 2000:6.1–6.30.

25. Johnston C, Carlson R, Tucker C, et al. Using BCMA software to improve patient safety in veterans administration medical centers. *J Health Inf Manag.* 2002:16(1):46–51.

26. Flynn E, Barker K, Carnahan B. National observational study of prescription dispensing accuracy and safety in 50 pharmacies. *J Am Pharm Assoc.* 2003;43(2): 191–200.

27. Quinlan P, Ashcroft D, Blenkinsopp A. Medication errors: a baseline survey of interventions recorded during the dispensing process in community pharmacies. *Int J Pharm Pract.* 2002;10(Suppl):R67.

28. Santell J, Cousins D, Hicks R. Medication error trends for 1999–2003. USP Drug Safety Review, Drug Topics Health System Edition. February 21, 2005, HSE22.

29. Lethal overdose claims third baby. CBS News. Indianapolis, IN, Sept 20, 2006. Available at: www.cbsnews.com/stories/2006/09/20/national/ main2026036.shtml? source=RSSattr=Health_2026036. Accessed August 2006.

30. Hospital makes another painkiller mistake. CBS News. Indianapolis, IN. Oct 16, 2006. Available at: www.cbsnews.com/stories/2006/10/16/health/main2091482. shtml?source=RSSattr=Health_2091482. Accessed August 2006.

31. Institute for Safe Medication Practices (ISMP). ISMP Medication Alert. May 2, 2001. Available at: www.ismp.org/Newsletters/acutecare/articles/20010502.asp?ptr=y. Accessed January 24, 2008.

32. Benfell C. *Fatal Errors: Hospitals Learn Lessons the Hard Way.* Santa Rosa, CA: American Iatrogenic Association; 1997. Available at: www.iatrogenic.org/fatalerr. html. Accessed January 24, 2008.

Chapter 2

Why Medication Incidents Occur

Objectives

After completing this chapter, the reader will be able to:

- Explain models and theories about human errors
- Describe studies investigating causes of medication incidents
- List classifications for types of errors
- List possible contributory factors to error

In order to prevent medication incidents from occurring, we need a full understanding of what an error is, what **causes** it, and what processes are involved. A number of theories have been put forth that explain what an error is and how it happens as well as how errors occur in relation to the medication use system. Various **contributory factors** have been suggested in order to identify where risks lie and promote the development of preventive strategies.

ERROR THEORY

The Person Approach versus the System Approach

James Reason, an international expert in the field of human error and systems analysis, has explained that error can be viewed from the "person approach" or the "system approach."[1] Traditionally, health professionals have approached the causes of error in personal terms, "naming, blaming, and shaming" the individuals involved (nurses, physicians, pharmacists, patients, etc.).[1] We tend to view the causes of unsafe acts to be human failings that lead to inattention, forgetfulness, negligence, and carelessness and assume that "bad things happen to bad people."[1] We attempt to address the issue through discipline, retraining, policies and procedures, and threats of litigation or, worse yet, sweeping it under the carpet and ignoring it.[1]

Although this personal approach is easy and sometimes convenient, it prevents the development of safe practices, since it does not identify causative factors or ways to prevent incidents from happening in the future. As a result, all too often, the very same incidents occur over and over again. Fear of punishment

13

created by this approach is one of the most damaging things contributing to medication incidents. Individuals will not report incidents if they are going to be reprimanded for them or report others for fear of retribution by coworkers for "tattling." If this happens, there are few opportunities to learn and develop preventive strategies to ensure these incidents do not occur again. And yet this continues to be a prevalent approach in pharmacies and health care generally.

In a study of subscribers to the safety publication "ISMP Medication Safety Alert" conducted by the U.S.-based Institute for Safe Medication Practices (ISMP) in June 2001, 15% of respondents said that not punishing someone for an error excuses poor performance and removes personal responsibility for patient safety.[2] Another 21% believed that lack of punishment might even increase carelessness—and that this would inhibit weeding out the "bad apples." Fortunately, only 9% of managers agreed with this view. According to the ISMP, terminating an employee in the wake of a fatal error or even for repeated errors is an "ineffective, emotionally charged knee-jerk reflex," which is far easier to do than getting to the bottom of an error and making system changes to make sure that it does not happen again.[2]

It is now recognized that a more constructive and effective approach to the issue of patient safety is what James Reason called the system approach.[1] It aims to understand how errors happen, determine the causative factors, and find solutions.

We have come to understand that errors are not just a result of human nature but rather are due to multiple contributory factors in the system. Humans are fallible and errors are to be expected. Reason has said that "it is often the best people who make the worst mistakes." He also observed that errors are not random but tend to be recurrent patterns, so that similar errors happen because the circumstances are the same, even if they involve different people.[1]

The "Accident Causation Model"

James Reason developed the Accident Causation Model, often also called the "Swiss Cheese Model" (Fig. 2.1), to depict how incidents happen.[1] It illustrates that systems have layers of barriers and defenses in place (e.g., people, forcing functions, labeling, procedures, and rules) but that there are still opportunities for failure, like holes in Swiss cheese. The holes are continually opening and shutting and shifting locations, but a circumstance can occur at any time where all the holes align by chance. When this happens, mistakes that would usually be caught are missed and the multilayered system fails, resulting in an incident.[1]

Reason further explains that the holes in the Swiss cheese arise because of **active failures** and **latent conditions**.[1] In the personal approach, the active failures are slips, lapses, mistakes, or procedural violations committed by people in the system, who are then blamed. The latent conditions exist within the system as a result of the design, procedures, or management. These latent conditions in the workplace include fatigue, understaffing, time pressure, inexperience, or inadequate equipment.[1] These weaknesses can lie dormant for many years before lining up with "active failures" of individuals in the system, resulting in an opportunity for an error to occur.[1]

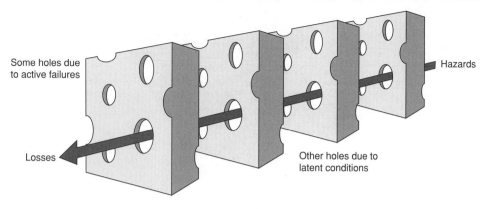

Some holes due to active failures

Hazards

Losses

Other holes due to latent conditions

Successive layers of defenses, barriers, and safeguards

FIGURE 2.1 James Reason's accident causation model, or the "Swiss cheese" model. (Adapted with permission from Reason J. Human error: models and management. *BMJ.* 2000;320:768–770.)

Since we cannot change human nature, which cause the active failures, the goal of error prevention and risk management should be to improve the structures and/or processes that make up the latent conditions so that **latent failures** are less likely to occur.[1] The task and the workplace should be targeted as well as the person.[1]

"Sharp- and Blunt-End" Model of Contributory Factors

Considering medication incidents from a systems analysis approach, we begin to understand that the causes of incidents go deeper than what occurred at the time of the event. The 2001 report on safety and quality of care entitled "Doing Less Harm," produced by the National Patient Safety Agency of the National Health Service (NHS) in Great Britain, depicts a model of the contributory factors to incidents that could be called a "sharp- and blunt-end" model (Fig. 2.2).[3] In concert with James Reason's systems approach, this model proposes that although incidents occur as a result of **immediate causes** at the "sharp end" of the drug delivery process, they are often a result of **root causes** at the "blunt end" of the system.[3,4] At the sharp end, contributory factors are more immediate and common causes involving active failures. They stem from factors in the environment and human errors by the health professional, patient, or caregiver and result in medication incidents for which individuals are usually blamed, as described by Reason in the "person approach."[1] These contributory factors have also been referred to as **proximal causes.**

At the blunt end of the medication delivery system, contributory factors involve root causes that are latent conditions related to the system of drug provision.[3] These may include the human factors, the drug or device manufacturer, the regulatory system, management, and organizational and institutional factors whose effects are not always apparent or seen immediately.

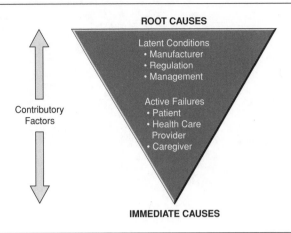

FIGURE 2.2 The "sharp- and blunt-end" model. (Source: National Health Service. Department of Health. National Patient Safety Agency. Doing less harm: improving the safety and quality of care through reporting, analysing and learning from adverse incidents involving NHS patients-key requirements for health care providers, August 2001 Available at: www.health.vic.gov.au/clinrisk/publications/doinglessharm.htm. Accessed January 24, 2008.)

These contributory factors have also been referred to as **system causes** or latent causes.

STUDIES OF CONTRIBUTORY FACTORS

Most studies of medication incidents and adverse events involving medications have focused on contributory factors at the sharp end of incident causation. Both hospital and voluntary reporting database studies describe common incidents. They show immediate errors occurring at every stage of the drug-use process.[5] Hospital studies identified the prescribing stage as most error-prone (56%), while reporting databases showed only 13% of reported errors from prescribing and the majority in drug administration.[5] Dose errors seemed to be the most common immediate drug therapy problems reported in hospital studies, whereas reporting databases showed wrong administration techniques to be most frequently reported.

The FDA 2001 adverse event analysis also reports common immediate causes of medication errors, classified according to the National Coordinating Council for Medication Errors Reporting and Prevention (NCC-MERP).[6] They report that an average of 19% of reports are caused by communication, 13% by name confusion, 20% by labeling, 42% by human factors, and 6% by packaging.[6]

Very few studies have reported the contributory factors that are root or system causes at the blunt end of incident causation.[5] Studies in hospitals have identified 16 different systems failures, the most common being dissemination of drug knowledge.[7] Knowledge deficits of pharmacotherapy were identified as the cause of 22% of errors, lack of information about the patients caused 14%, and memory slips and lapses caused 9%.[7]

The U.S.-based Institute for Safe Medication Practices (ISMP) reviewed thousands of reports of medication incidents from the U.S. Pharmacopeia Medication Errors Reporting Program (USP MER) and the U.S. Food and Drug Administration's MedWatch Program; it visited hundreds of related Web sites and found that contributory factors in all cases were multifactoral.[8] They also found that all incidents involved similar circumstances that generally can be reduced to a relatively small number of common immediate causes and root causes. [8]

CLASSIFICATION OF CONTRIBUTORY FACTORS

Based on the models and theories of error and research into medication incidents, contributory factors to medication incidents can be classified into a number of categories that fall into the broader categories of common immediate causes and root causes.

The most frequent immediate or common causes have been identified in the general categories summarized in Table 2.1. They involve occurrences during the prescribing, preparation, delivery, and administration of the medication, generally the responsibility of an individual (e.g., pharmacist, physician, technician, nurse).

Contributory root or system causes are summarized in Table 2.2. They include a number of ways in which the system can fail, right from a drug's production to its administration to the individual patient. This involves individuals as well as health care organizations (institutions or community pharmacy chains), government approval bodies, and the pharmaceutical industry.[4,9]

IMMEDIATE OR COMMON CAUSES OF MEDICATION INCIDENTS

Factors that have been identified as immediate or common causes are described briefly here. They are discussed in further detail in the following chapters, along with examples and preventive strategies.

TABLE 2.1
Immediate or Active Causes of Medication Incidents

- Failed communication
- Calculation errors
- Drug and drug-device problems
- Incorrect drug administration by health professionals or by patients
- Lack of patient counseling and education

TABLE 2.2
Root or System Causes

- Human factors
- Dispensing process
- Pharmacy workload
- Environment
- Organizational issues
- Manufacturing issues
- Technology

Failed Communication

The communication of the prescription order from physician through to the patient involves many steps and opportunities for error. These may include misread handwriting, confusion of similar (sound-alike and look-alike, or "SALAD") drug names, fax errors, missing information, ambiguous or incomplete prescriptions, inappropriate use of symbols and abbreviations, and poor verbal communication.

Written communication can be misinterpreted owing to unclear numbers, poor placement of zeros and decimal points or their omission, use of metric and apothecary systems of stating measures, misinterpretation of abbreviations, and ambiguous or incomplete orders.[9–11] Handwritten communications, in particular, can cause confusion, more so if there are similar named drugs and if they have same route and dose (e.g., tramadol 50 mg and trazodone 50 mg). A variety of written figures can result in misinterpretation of prescription orders, particularly zeros and decimal points (e.g., name and number can run together, as when Inderal20 is interpreted as Inderal 120).[9–11]

Ambiguous or incomplete orders can also lead to incidents; for example, an order seemed to be written for "Ativan 25 mg"; the pharmacist, recognizing that this drug did not come in that strength, thought it must mean "Ativan 2.5 mg" when it actually was meant to be "Atarax 25 mg."

Abbreviations and short forms are a huge source of error because there is poor standardization. Although there are accepted Latin abbreviations, some of these may be idiosyncratic.[9–11] Short forms for drug names and prescription directions can lead to serious errors because of multiple meanings, misinterpretation, and misreading[10,11] (e.g., "DPH" can be interpreted as diphenhydramine, an antihistamine, or diphenylhydantoin, an antiseizure medication; both come as 50-mg dosage forms).[9]

A frequent problem with written and verbal prescriptions is drugs with similar names (SALAD), which caused 13% of errors reported to the FDA in 2001 (e.g., Zantac and Zyrtec).[9–11] This sort of thing is more likely to cause an incident when the product is new and the pharmacist is not familiar with it because of "confirmation bias" (discussed further in Chapter 4).

In addition, verbal communication between health professionals and between the health professional and patient, in person or on the telephone, can be misunderstood. Accents, dialects, pronunciations, and background noise contribute to confusion in verbal orders, and people often assume that they heard correctly and do not verify.

There is also huge potential for miscommunication with the patient, including:

- Patient name mix ups: for example, Mr. Reimer was confused with Mr. Westheimer and received the wrong prescription.[12]
- Language issues cause errors where English is a second language or is misheard.
- Misunderstandings or ambiguous requests: for example, the patient requests, "my heart pills," which could be one of several prescriptions on file.

Calculation Errors

Critical errors can occur in calculating doses, particularly for pediatric patients and in the case of intravenous medications (which can include calculations of dose by weight and reconstitution calculations). Such errors may be due to poor arithmetic, decimal point errors, or misunderstanding of the label directions—sometimes resulting in grave errors of 10-fold or more doses. Also, various dosing algorithms are available, and either the algorithm can be miscalculated or a different algorithm than the one intended may be used. These types of errors occur repeatedly even when multiple checks are made by different people.[6–9]

Problems Related to Drugs and Drug Devices

Drug and drug device–related problems contribute to the occurrence of a variety of medication errors.[13] Defective labeling accounted for 20% of errors reported to the FDA in 2001.[6] Some errors occur when such labeling is not seen or is misinterpreted (e.g., labeling not on inner wrapper and package discarded). Other labeling errors involve mixups of drugs with labels of similar color or design.

Drug devices such as infusion pumps, automatic intravenous compounders, or counting machines can result in errors due to misuse, poor maintenance, or failure of the device. For example, infusion pumps have been the source of several types of incidents, including dosing errors that occurred because of incorrect programming (e.g., 705 mL/hr was programmed instead of 7.5).[13]

Incorrect Drug Administration

Even when the medication has left the pharmacy, there are numerous opportunities for incidents to occur during administration, including use of the wrong route, incorrect frequency of administration or missed dose, and incorrect dose.

In the hospital, several people may be involved in drug administration and misunderstandings may occur. Sometimes these incidents involve medication administered by the wrong route (e.g., intravenously [IV] instead of intramuscularly [IM], eardrops given to the eye, topical liquid taken orally, or oral liquid given IV when an oral syringe is mistaken for an intravenous syringe). This has resulted in tragic consequences, as when an intravenous vinca alkaloid product (vincristine, vinblastine) has been administered intrathecally. This has occurred repeatedly, despite warnings, and results in immediate death due to brain damage.[14]

In the community, the patient or caregiver may inadvertently commit an error, usually by administering an over- or underdose or giving a drug at an incorrect frequency (e.g., interpreting thrice daily dosing of an antibiotic as meaning during waking hours only). Although pharmacists are not present for these errors, they can help to prevent them through patient education.

Lack of Patient Counseling and Education

As noted above, lack of communication between the health professional and the patient can result in many kinds of medication incidents. However, even when verbal or written communication occurs, there may be misunderstandings about the purpose of a medication, dosing time, route, and amount. Changes in medication or dosing may not be known by the patient, and assumptions may be made about the patient's level of knowledge and understanding or ability to understand and comply.

Pharmacists find it difficult to accept responsibility for these types of incidents because they do not go home with the patient. However, there is one major step in the medication provision process that may have been omitted by the pharmacist in such a case: patient counseling and education. In fact, lack of patient education may be the ultimate cause of medication discrepancies becoming incidents, since patient counseling gives the pharmacist a final opportunity to catch many of the types of problems discussed above. Any misunderstandings can be brought to light and clarified during counseling. Patients who are adequately educated about the purpose of their medications will be more likely to understand how to administer them. Also, any changes in the patient's dose or strength of medication can be noted during counseling, as some physicians may not properly inform their patients or the patients may not remember or understand what the doctor said. The pharmacist also has the opportunity during counseling to show the medication to the patient as a final check that the correct medication has been dispensed.

ROOT OR SYSTEM CAUSES OF MEDICATION INCIDENTS

Factors that have been identified as root or system causes are described briefly below. They are discussed in further detail in the following chapters, along with examples and preventive strategies.

Human Factors

It is now understood that the immediate causes of the errors discussed above combine with various **human factors**, including psychological and physiological factors that prevent the detection of errors or cause them to occur. Pharmacists as well as technicians, physicians, nurses, and patients are all subject to these types of influences.

Diversion of attention is something that pharmacists are very familiar with because they have many distractions in the course of the day; these are environmental in nature—noise, heat, motion.[15,16]

Physiological factors such as fatigue, sleep loss, alcohol, drugs, illness, hunger, and even the simple need for a bathroom break may distract the pharmacist or cause him or her to be less attentive, leading to errors.[17]

Similarly, psychological factors—including emotional states such as boredom, frustration, anxiety, and anger—can lead to errors. These may be triggered by internal or external factors such as overwork, interpersonal relationships, and other forms of stress.[16]

Difficulties in finding the solutions to problems and problems of perception also work at the psychological level to contribute to the occurrence of incidents.[17] The individual pharmacist's perceptions may be related to incidents because they create mental tension and distractions, which may lead to a breakdown in cognitive functioning.[17] These perceptions may include the following[16]:

- Poor relationships with supervisors
- Overall job dissatisfaction
- Perception that breaks are inadequate
- Impulsive and field-dependent personality (reduced ability to focus and attend to details)
- Sleep deprivation
- Perception that ambient lighting and equipment are inadequate

Lack of knowledge about a patient, equipment, or new drug can be at the root of many adverse effects (e.g., a potential drug interaction with a new medication may not be recognized).[9]

Lack of knowledge of course can also apply to the prescriber, who may confuse names and dosages, be unaware of drug interactions or contraindications, etc., and the patient, who may commit errors in administration through lack of knowledge about the medications he or she is using, again making it critical to educate the patient.

Dispensing Processes and Drug Distribution

The multitude of problems described above that occur at the "sharp end" of the medication use process point to problems in the dispensing process. Since the dispensing process involves many steps and possibly many different individuals working in a sometimes difficult environment (see below), there are many points at which things can go wrong and contribute to an incident—from improper storage of medications, misselection of a drug from storage, computer entry errors, miscounting, and so forth.[18] Distractions, lack of organization (see below), poor environment, miscommunication, and poor awareness of possible pitfalls all contribute.[19]

Work Schedules and Workload

Health care workers often believe that overwork is the cause of adverse incidents, but this is a debated issue. There may be an optimal workload level below which more errors are likely to occur, but they can also occur above that level.[16] There is no doubt that if workers are rushed, fatigued, and stressed or unhappy, as discussed above, errors are more likely to be made.

Technology and Equipment Design

Well-designed technology and equipment can help to prevent errors, but poor training, improper use, and poor maintenance can cause these factors to contribute to an incident.

Computer design and errors in software programs that provide incorrect information or fail to update information—for example, in drug interaction alerts—can affect incident rates. Dispensing systems, such as those providing unit doses, have great potential to reduce errors in administration, but errors can occur in labeling and quality control for packaging. Because unit-dose dispensers generally supply 24 hours of medication at a time, errors that do occur are at least not perpetuated for more than 24 hours. Electronic prescribing has been promoted to reduce prescribing errors by avoiding legibility issues, providing prompts for dosage and frequency and drug interactions; however overreliance on computer prompts and poor training of practitioners in the use of programs can contribute to errors.

Robots are more frequently being installed to reduce the chance for human error; however, there is still a human element, as someone has to interpret and input orders and administer medications. Therefore, one cannot become overreliant on technology.

The design of all these technologies is critical because they must take into account the humans who work with them as well as the possible software and hardware problems. For example, an ISMP report described an incident resulting from a faulty keyboard with a malfunctioning "m" key, resulting in two order entry errors where "mg" became just "g" on medication administration records. Luckily this was detected before a 1,000-fold overdose occurred.[20]

Environment

Various factors in the environment can cause distractions or contribute to human error, affecting an individual's problem-solving ability and stress level.[15,19] Poor design of the physical environment, work area organization, and equipment (e.g., noisy printers and telephones) can contribute to distractions and stress. Work areas often have inadequate storage areas, clutter, or insufficient space for work (counters and walking areas); there are also frequent interruptions. The noise, heat, lighting, color, and physical barriers in the pharmacy environment must also be considered.[15,19]

Organizations

Organizations such as hospitals and chain pharmacies can contribute to errors by lack of attention to the issues outlined above. A number of obstacles in organizations such as hospitals and pharmacies may contribute to systemic causes of medication incidents. For a start, the systems involving medication use in any organization are complex: there are multiple individuals involved and multiple stakeholders; the system for ordering, dispensing, and administering medications involves many people, including physicians, nurses, pharmacists, clerks, technicians, and patients; there are multiple decisions to be made involving drugs, names, routes, and doses; and there are many communications, both written and verbal.[18] This complexity can also result in poor access to information about patients and faulty knowledge about drugs and the potential for error.[7]

Within organizations, individuals and their idiosyncrasies (such as the use of nonstandard abbreviations, as discussed above) are often tolerated and customary ways of doing things that may contribute to error can be difficult to challenge or to alter.

When it comes to addressing the issue of medication incidents, there is often a lack of ownership for problems involving the whole system. In addition, the "blame and shame" approach discussed earlier is often predominant, so that individuals are less likely to report an error and error management is often limited to "damage control" and punishment rather than discovery of contributory factors and future prevention.

An organization's staffing and scheduling policies can also be at fault. As mentioned above, a shift in rate of work is most likely to contribute to incidents, so staffing that does not reflect changes in work demands throughout the day, long shifts, or too many continuous days without any break can contribute to incidents.

An organization is also responsible for the training of staff involved in the medication management process—receiving orders, order transcribing, selecting drugs, to inputting orders, giving out medication, and administration/oversight. Although these seem like simple tasks, they can contribute to incidents if staff is not appropriately trained in safe processes and risk reduction.

In addition, many organizations do not have a **culture of patient safety.** This involves an awareness of errors and the things we have discussed thus far as well as a commitment to the prevention of error and the promotion and improvement of patient safety—that is, a systems approach as opposed to individual blame. If patient safety is not actively worked toward through all aspects of the organization, there is a good chance that errors will happen and continue to happen. This is discussed further in later chapters.

The risk of incidents is likely to be higher if an organization does not conduct analyses of risk to determine where errors might occur, if they have a policy or plan that causes or potentially causes incidents, and if changes need to be made in the system. The analysis of risk and root-cause analysis are discussed in the following chapters.

Health care organizations, regulatory bodies, and provincial and federal governments also play a part. They must be involved in creating barriers to medication incidents, setting standards, and implementing state and organization-wide systems with a view to promoting patient safety.

The Drug Development Process

When we follow medication incidents to the root, we sometimes find problems in the product development process and the health care industry, particularly drug product labeling and naming. Examples of this include:

- Same-color labeling of different drugs by the same company
- New drugs named with names that are very similar to those of other drugs, including brand name suffixes like XL or SL
- Unclearly marked dosages

In a recent article titled "Lessons lost by the global pharmaceutical industry," the Institute for Safe Medication Practices (ISMP) noted that the FDA and U.S. pharmaceutical companies have responded to the evidence on errors caused by packaging and naming of pharmaceuticals and have made some changes, such as changing Losec to Prilosec to avoid confusion with Lasix and adding a warning label to vinca alkaloids stating "FATAL if given intrathecally. IV USE ONLY." However, this was only done in the United States; in Canada and the United Kingdom, there continue to be errors and fatalities as a result of this confusion.[21]

Organizations such as the ISMP, governments, and regulatory authorities must work together with the pharmaceutical industry to be proactive in carrying actions taken in the United States and other countries as well as in identifying potential errors in packaging design and the naming of new products. There are many barriers to this, including regulatory issues and the cost of necessary changes.

SUMMARY

The contributory factors introduced in this chapter will be discussed in greater detail in later chapters.

It is important to keep in mind that most incidents involve more than one contributory cause, usually both root and immediate common causes. Risk management and preventive strategies that take contributory causes into account are discussed in the next chapter.

Reflective Questions

1. List and explain the various theories relating to error and medication incidents.
2. Discuss three contributory factors to medication incidents involving immediate causes.
3. Discuss two communication issues in the pharmacy that can contribute medication incidents.
4. Discuss three contributory factors to medication incidents involving root causes.

REFERENCES

1. Reason J. Human error: models and management. *BMJ*. 2000;320:768–770.
2. Institute for Safe Medication Practices (ISMP) ISMP survey on perceptions of a non-punitive culture nets some surprising results. ISMP Medication Safety Alert. August 22, 2001. Available at: www.ismp.org/MSAarticles/nonpunitive.html. Accessed July 7, 2004.
3. National Health Service, Department of Health. National Patient Safety Agency. Doing less harm: improving the safety and quality of care through reporting, analyzing and learning from adverse incidents involving NHS patients-key requirements for health care providers. August 2001. Available at: www.health.vic.gov.au/clinrisk/publications/doinglessharm.htm. Accessed January 24, 2008.
4. National Steering Committee on Patient Safety. Building a safer system—a national integrated strategy for improving patient safety in Canadian health care. September 2002. Available at: www.pharmacists.ca/content/about_cpha/whats_happening/cpha_in_action/pdf/PatientSafetyBuildingSaferSystemReport_Sept02.pdf. Accessed February 2008.
5. Kanjanarat P, Winterstein, Johns T, et al. Nature of preventable adverse drug events in hospitals: a literature review. *Am J Health Syst Pharm*. 2003;60(14): 1750–1759.
6. Thomas M, Holquist C, Phillips J. Med error reports to FDA show a mixed bag. FDA safety page. *Drug Topics*. 2001;1:23. Available at: www.fda.gov/cder/drug/MedErrors/mixed.pdf. Accessed June 2006.
7. Leape LL, Bates DW, Cullen J, et al. The ADE Prevention Study Group. Systems analysis of adverse drug events. *JAMA*. 1995;274(1):35–43.
8. Cohen M. Causes of medication errors. In: Cohen M, ed. *Medication Errors—Causes, Prevention and Risk Management*. Boston: Jones and Bartlett; 2000:1.1–1.7.
9. U.S. Food and Drug Administration. Center for Drug Evaluation and Research. Medication Errors. Available at: www.fda.gov/cder/drug/MedErrors/default.htm. Accessed July 2006.
10. Institute for Safe Medication Practices (ISMP). Special Issue. Don't use these dangerous abbreviations or dose designations. Available at: www.ismp.or/ MSAarticles/specialissuetable.html. Accessed April 18, 2002.
11. Institute for Safe Medication Practices (ISMP). List of error-prone abbreviations, symbols and dose designations. Available at: www.ismp.org/Tools/errorproneabbreviations.pdf. Accessed September 13, 2006.
12. Stewart I. Focus on error prevention. *Pharm Connect*. 2002;9(2):46.

13. Institute for Safe Medication Practices (ISMP). High alert drugs and infusion pumps: extra precautions required. *Can Saf Bull.* 2004;4(4):2.
14. Abraham C. Dosage errors imperil children: study. *Globe and Mail.* April 11, 2002.
15. Caverly WM. The seaworthy vessel—attractive practice environment. Presentation at CPhA Conference 2001, Halifax, NS, May 2001.
16. Grasha A. Misconceptions about pharmacy workload. *CPJ.* 2001;134(3):26–35.
17. Grasha A. Psychosocial factors, workload and risk of medication errors. *US Pharm.* 1996;21:96–109. Available at: www.uspharmacist.com/oldformat.asp? url=newlook/files/Feat/MedicationErrors.htm&pub_id.8&article_id=859. Accessed September 2006.
18. Institute for Safe Medication Practices (ISMP). Frequently asked questions. Available at: www.ismp.org/faq.asp. Accessed January 24, 2008.
19. Grissinger M. Insights into human nature can improve our safety systems. P&T, 2004;29(12):748, 751. Available at: www.ptcommunity.com/ptjournal/fulltext/29/12/PTJ2912748.pdf. Acessed September 2006.
20. Institute for Safe Medication Practices (ISMP). ISMP medication safety alert. ISPM Newsletter, 2002;7(8):4.
21. Institute for Safe Medication Practices (ISMP). Lessons lost by the global pharmaceutical industry. Medication safety articles. Available at www.ismp.or/MSAarticles/GlobalPharm.html. Accessed April 18, 2002.

Chapter 3

Prevention of Medication Incidents: Risk Management to Improve Patient Safety

Objectives

After completing this chapter, the reader will be able to:

- Describe the elements involved in risk management for pharmacy
- List at least three organizations involved currently in issues involving medical and medication safety
- List strategies that organizations and individuals can take to prevent or reduce the risk of medication incidents

Now that we understand the complexity of medication incidents, with their multiple immediate and root causes, we can consider ways of preventing or at least reducing and managing the risk of such incidents and improving patient safety.

Risk management comprises those administrative and clinical activities that aim to identify, reduce, and evaluate the chance of injury or loss to individuals and the organization.[1,2] There are two components to risk management.[3] One involves activities to limit the incidence of dangerous incidents by preventing them from occurring. Since this will never be wholly effective because of the complexity of systems and human elements, a second component of risk management must involve efforts to moderate the medication use system so that it is better able to tolerate the occurrence of medication incidents and to limit their damaging effects.[3]

Measures to prevent or reduce the risk of medication incidents must involve all members and parts of the system, including providers, patients, leaders, purchasers, industry, regulatory and professional bodies, licensing and accreditation bodies, and finally academic institutions that train health care professionals.[4]

ELEMENTS OF RISK MANAGEMENT IN PHARMACY

When organizations prepare to take action to prevent or reduce medication incidents, they embark on significant work that must be approached systematically. The elements of risk management in relation to pharmacy include a series of activities, as illustrated in Figure 3.1, including preventive strategies, continuous quality improvement, incident reports, and root cause analysis.

The first element of risk management in pharmacy is prevention strategies. These can be put into place at many levels in the system, including those involving the whole system, general strategies for organizations, and more specific strategies that can be put in place by individual pharmacists, pharmacy technicians, nurses, physicians, and patients.

Another element of risk management in pharmacy is the process of **continuous quality improvement (CQI).** This involves using various tools such as **risk analysis** to analyze the potential risks in a system and **failure modes effect analysis (FMEA)** to evaluate new products and identify and prevent potential product and process problems before they occur.

Regular self-assessment by pharmacists of their practices is another important part of CQI in pharmacy. This can be used by individual pharmacists for self-improvement or by the whole pharmacy organization (pharmacy department in an institution, a pharmacy chain, or an independent community pharmacy), leading to the development of a **patient safety plan** for the pharmacy.

An effective incident reporting system is also a critical element of risk management in pharmacy, so that when an incident does occur, lessons can be learned by all involved. This should be done internally in the organization or pharmacy where an incident occurs as well as through a national reporting system, so that all pharmacists and others involved in the system can learn and develop strategies for future prevention.

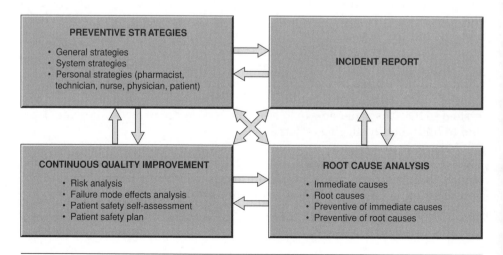

FIGURE 3.1 Elements of Risk Management for Medication Incidents.

In order to develop strategies for future prevention, a **root cause analysis** should be conducted following the incident to identify all immediate and root causes and to devise the strategies and actions that must be taken to prevent the occurrence of similar incidents in the future.

Each of these elements is discussed here or in later chapters. The handling of a medication incident, including incident reporting and root cause analysis (analysis of immediate and root causes and preventive strategies for those causes), is discussed in Chapter 8. Continuous quality improvement by pharmacists and pharmacies through risk analysis and pharmacy/pharmacist self-assessment and the development of a patient safety plan is discussed in Chapter 9. Specific preventive strategies for immediate and root causes are discussed in detail in Chapters 4 to 7. The remainder of this chapter discusses prevention strategies for the system, organizations, and individuals.

SYSTEM PREVENTIVE STRATEGIES

After patient safety issues were brought into awareness by the various reports and studies discussed in Chapter 1, there was an explosion of initiatives from governments and organizations designed to deal with them. Some efforts are directed toward raising awareness and educating both professionals and the public about these issues and preventive strategies, while other initiatives document errors and recommend changes and preventive strategies in response to specific types of errors. Most involve patient safety in the medical system as a whole, including medication safety, while a few focus solely on the latter.

Organizations and Activities Involving Patient Safety

Appendix A lists the various organizations in the United States involved in medical and medication safety, incident prevention and analysis, and some of the activities they engage in to improve patient safety. There are similar organizations either existing or being developed in other countries, such as the Canadian Patient Safety Institute (CPSI), which is conducting research and developing an incident reporting system; the National Patient Safety Agency (NPSA) in the United Kingdom, which has a mandatory incident reporting program for hospital and primary care; and the Australian Patient Safety Foundation (APSF), which has a voluntary reporting program for hospitals.[5]

Government Action

Following the Institute of Medicine report entitled *To Err is Human: Building a Safer Health System*, President Bill Clinton signed an executive order requiring federal agencies and departments to develop, within 90 days, a list of activities to make patient care safer. This has resulted in a number of new programs at numerous U.S. agencies.[6]

Some legislation and guidelines have been enacted in the United States since then to ensure that responsibility is accepted for patient safety and measures are taken to prevent errors. Legislative efforts include the federal Patient Safety and Quality Improvement Act of 2005, signed into law in July, 2005.[7,8] It sets the stage for improved reporting of patient safety information by assuring confidentiality and legal protection of information collected and shared with patient safety organizations and will certify a number of organizations to collect patient safety information and submit it to a national patient safety database for research.[7,8] The FDA has also proposed regulations calling for bar coding on medications and blood products and new pharmaceutical industry requirements for reporting medication safety issues to the FDA.[7]

A number of states, including California, Texas, and Florida, have passed regulations or statutes that require a quality assurance program for each hospital and community pharmacy in their state, and many states have implemented quality assurance programs to reduce errors in pharmacy practice.[9,10]

Recommendations for System Changes to Prevent Medication Incidents in the United States

The U.S. Institute of Medicine (IOM) released a report in 2006 entitled *Preventing Medication Errors,* which made recommendations to affect system changes, many of which had been recommended previously by other organizations.[11] Significant recommendations included the following:

- A shift from studying incidence rates to the development and validation of error-prevention strategies.
- All prescribers and pharmacies should be using e-prescriptions by 2010.
- Specific strategies for consumers and providers to strengthen their partnership and provide better consumer-oriented drug information.
- Importance of communicating clinical information among all who need it including community pharmacists.
- Improve error reporting through promotion by all stakeholders of reporting initially to the USP-ISMP Medication Error Reporting Program (MERP).
- Pharmacy licensing boards should require community pharmacy safety initiatives including quality improvement activities.
- Academic accreditation agencies should set new standards requiring professional schools to provide safety education.
- The FDA, the pharmaceutical industry, and others must work together to eliminate medical product errors through actions to address labeling and packaging issues.

GENERAL PREVENTIVE STRATEGIES FOR ORGANIZATIONS

Although the strategies discussed above should affect the whole system involved in medication use, it is generally within organizations that the changes must take place. Health care organizations such as institutions, pharmacy chains, and health districts must take the lead in implementing system changes to improve patient safety. They must show clear organizational responsibility and accountability for patient safety. And they must review and manage patient safety concerns within the organizations.[12]

The Institute for Healthcare Improvement (IHI) notes that organizations that have been most successful in reducing harm have made changes in four key areas: developing a culture of safety, reducing harm from high-hazard medications, improving medication core processes (ordering, dispensing, and administering), and improving medication reconciliation.[13]

Developing a Culture of Safety

In addressing the issue of patient safety, the United States, the UK, and Canada have all noted that building a safety culture is the first step to improving patient safety.[14] The concept and importance of a **culture of safety** comes from high-risk industries such as nuclear power.[14] It is defined as "an integrated pattern of individual and organizational behavior, based upon shared beliefs and values, that continuously seeks to minimize patient harm which may result from the processes of care delivery."[1]

The following have been identified as elements of a patient safety culture[15]:

• Commitment to safety by leadership
• Resources for patient safety
• Safety versus production is a priority
• Open and effective communication
• Openness about problems and errors
• The organization learns from errors
• Tracking of unsafe acts

In particular, there must be an atmosphere of mutual trust whereby staff members can talk freely about safety problems and how to solve them without fear of blame or punishment.[13]

There has been some success in using training to improve patient safety. In one study, nurses in clinical leadership roles received a presentation on the rate of adverse events in health care, theoretical models of human error, how to learn from errors, teamwork, and safety leadership. Compared with a control group, there was a significant improvement from before the training to 10 months later in perceptions about safety.[16]

Reducing Harm from High-Hazard Medications

It has been observed that error prevention efforts are more effective when they are focused on specific high-hazard medications or error-prone situations.[17] The ISMP regularly updates a list of **high-alert drugs,** defined as "drugs that bear a heightened risk of causing significant patient harm when they are used in error."[18]

High-alert drugs should be identified, along with potential errors that might occur with them, and then measures put in place to prevent errors. Techniques should be developed to simplify and standardize the process for ordering, preparing, and administering these drugs.[19] Specific recommendation have been made by IHI on reducing adverse events involving anticoagulants, insulin, narcotics and sedatives, chemotherapy, electrolytes, antibiotics, and intravenous medications (see Appendix B).[13]

Improving Medication Core Processes

To Err is Human, the U.S. report on patient safety, recommended system strategies specific to medication processes.[20] They include the following:

- Standardizing prescription writing and prescribing
- Utilizing unit-dose systems
- Utilizing prescribing software to end handwritten prescriptions
- Utilizing dispensing software that allows system checks (e.g., flagging for irregular dosing and similar drug names)
- Instituting special procedures and protocols for high-risk medications

The ISMP has identified "ten key elements of the medication use system" that most often affect the medication use process and describes the medication errors associated with them (see Table 3.1).[21] These form the basis of the pharmacy/pharmacist assessment process devised by ISMP, which is discussed further in Chapter 9.

As data have been accumulated through various reporting systems about the most common and critical types of errors, preventive strategies have been

---

TABLE 3.1
ISMP's 10 Key Elements of a Safe Medication Use System

1. Patient information when prescribing, dispensing, administering
2. Accurate and accessible drug information for all health professionals
3. Verification of drug information and removing communication barriers
4. Proper drug, packaging labeling and nomenclature, and unit dose dispensing
5. Standardizing drug dosage and administration times and drug storage in patient areas
6. Safety assessment of drug delivery devices and independent double-checks during use
7. Well-designed systems with attention to environmental factors
8. Staff education and competence
9. Ongoing patient education on medication use and patient safety
10. Processes to improve quality and risk management to detect and correct errors before they reach patients

Source: Institute for Safe Medication Practices. Frequently asked questions. Available at: www.ismp.org/faq.asp#Question_9/. Accessed September 20, 2007.

developed by various organizations for specific types of errors. These are listed in Appendix B, and many are discussed in later chapters of this book.

Improving Medication Reconciliation

Medication reconciliation is "the process of creating the most accurate list possible of all medications a patient is taking—including drug name, dosage, frequency, and route—and comparing that list against the physician's admission, transfer, and/or discharge orders."[13] The goal is to provide correct medications to the patient at all transition points within the health care institution.[13] Failed communication about a patient's medication during vulnerable transition points in the continuum of health care, including admission, transfers between care settings, and discharge, contributes to as many as 50% of all medication errors and up to 20% of adverse drug events in hospitals.[22]

In 2005, the Joint Commission on Health Care made it a major safety goal to require hospitals, ambulatory care, assisted living, behavioral health, home care, and long-term-care organizations to reconcile medications across the continuum of care by January 2006.[22] Except in emergency or urgent situations, this involves obtaining an accurate list of current patient prescriptions and over-the-counter, herbal, and dietary supplements (dose, route, frequency, indication, time of last dose) prior to administering the first dose of medications.[22,23] This list should be gathered through a medication history and reviewed by the prescriber, who then prescribes admission medications. The list is compared with admission medications within 24 hours of admission and discrepancies are resolved. This list is reviewed and compared with new orders each time the patient is transferred to a different level of care and when he or she is discharged. It is communicated to the next provider of service, the patient's primary care physician, and the patient, who is encouraged to share it with his or her pharmacy. A weakness in this process is the lack of involvement of the community pharmacy, which is not generally part of the formal process but rather engaged only through the patient's direction.

PREVENTIVE STRATEGIES FOR PHARMACIES

Preventive strategies specific to reducing medication incidents have been proposed for hospitals and for distribution processes in both hospital or ambulatory pharmacies.

Hospital Pharmacy Preventive Strategies

U.S. and Canadian hospital pharmacist organizations have put forth system strategies specific to reducing medication incidents in hospitals.[24,25] They recommend that the pharmacy and therapeutics (P&T) committee (composed of pharmacists, physicians, nurses, and other health professionals) should be responsible for formulating policies regarding the evaluation, selection, and therapeutic uses of drugs. Partnerships between individuals, professions, and organizations must be developed to address operational/ systemic deficiencies that may contribute to medication-related events. Pharmacists should be involved in the development of organizational policies regarding procedures, protocols, and guidelines pertaining to pharmaceuticals. This will promote consistent and accurate processes for drug prescribing, administration, and storage, particularly for high-alert drugs. Specific recommendations are discussed in the following sections with regard to the needed policies, pharmacists' responsibilities, and best practices within hospitals.

Policies Needed

Policies should be developed in the hospital or health care institution regarding the following[24,25]:

- Efficient and safe distribution of medications (see best practices, below)
- Hiring and assigning personnel who have been adequately trained, supervised, and evaluated
- Sufficient personnel with reasonable workload levels and working hours to perform tasks adequately
- The work environment for the preparation of drug products should be suitable to reduce sources of error, such as frequent interruptions
- Clear lines of authority and areas of responsibility for medication ordering, dispensing, and administration systems
- Quality improvement and peer review programs with respect to safe medication use, including formal drug-use evaluation of high-alert drugs
- Mechanism to collect and evaluate medication error reports, investigate causes of errors, and develop programs for decreasing their occurrence
- Appropriate clinical information about patients accessible to pharmacists and others processing drug orders
- Adequate drug information resources accessible to all health care providers
- Technological innovations, such as bar coding, unit dose packaging, computerized physician order entry (CPOE), automated dispensing machines (ADM), and computerized medication administration records, installed in hospital pharmacies (see Chapter 7 for discussion of these).

Pharmacist Responsibilities

Pharmacists working in institutions should have the following responsibilities[24,25]:

- Provision of all sterile and nonsterile drug products used within the organization by 24-hour or "on-call" service
- Maintenance of medication profiles for all patients
- Conducting of drug order reviews to evaluate the appropriateness of the orders and identify potential problems before orders are dispensed

- Involvement in direct patient-care activities such as ward-based pharmaceutical care, pharmacist-managed or collaborative drug therapy programs, patient education, and seamless care activities
- Provision and routine inspection of floor-stock medications for urgent medication orders
- Counseling of patients on discharge
- Education programs conducted in conjunction with nursing and the medical staff regarding risk management, medication errors, their causes, and methods of prevention

Best Practices

Within the hospital or institution, the following practices should be observed[24,25]:

- Unit-dose drug distribution and control system
- List of standard abbreviations
- Standard drug concentrations and dosage charts and drug administrations times
- Adequate storage, labeling, packaging, and product integrity of floor-stock medication
- Adequate written and oral communication; review and verification or original orders and documentation
- Avoiding use of patient's own or "home" medications
- Providing discharged patients only with labeled drug products according to regulations

Ambulatory Pharmacy Preventive Strategies

Preventive strategies in ambulatory pharmacy generally fall within the responsibility of individual pharmacists and are, therefore, discussed in part in the following section on personal preventive strategies. However, many ambulatory pharmacies are owned and/or operated by organizations, which set policies, and are influenced by the culture of the organization, as discussed above. They are therefore in a position to set policies and provide tools for use within ambulatory pharmacies that can prevent or reduce medication incidents. Such measures would include the following[9]:

- Provide pharmacy software that is designed using forcing functions and constraints that make it virtually impossible to make certain kinds of errors; for example, pertinent patient information must be entered before an order can be complete, alerts are triggered by drug duplicates or look-alike sound-alike medications
- Provide software that screens for duplicate drug therapies, patient allergies, potential drug interactions, and dose ranges; also have policies that require pharmacists to document the handling of computer alerts resulting from screening.

- Institute automation where possible, such as bar-coding and dispensing machines, and ensure proper training of individuals regarding their use.
- Provide an up-to-date library and drug information search capability.
- Ensure that work areas are designed for good work flow and minimal distractions.
- Provide sufficient well-trained staff and allow for appropriate length of shifts and smooth workloads.
- Require documentation, patient monitoring, patient counseling, and patient education.
- Require independent double-check systems so that individuals check one another's work.
- Have policies and processes for pharmacists and technicians to self-document medication errors and near misses and an anonymous system for reporting, handling, and discussing these both within each pharmacy and the entire organization.
- Encourage and allow for the continuing education of pharmacists and technicians.
- Require Failure Modes Effects Analysis (FMEA) of new products and procedures in the pharmacy.

Many of these issues are discussed in more detail in following chapters.

PERSONAL PREVENTIVE STRATEGIES

Although it is clear that contributory factors to medication incidents are multifactoral, including both root and immediate causes, and that blame should never be ascribed to one individual, individuals do have a role to play in preventing medication incidents and promoting safe medication practices. However, some of these measures are clearly beyond the scope of individuals; for example, changing the name of a drug like Losec so that it will never be confused with Lasix. Nevertheless, individuals do have opportunities to play a role within organizations, as discussed above, and through personal practices and actions. The following sections describe measures that can be adopted by individual pharmacists, pharmacy technicians, nurses, physicians, and patients to prevent medication incidents.

Prevention by Individuals in Organizations

While the above strategies involving the system may be beyond the power of individual pharmacists to enact, pharmacists can lobby for these system changes through pharmacy advocacy organizations or other bodies. Pharmacists are often in positions within organizations to influence some of these things by[20]:

- Providing leadership
- Respecting human limits in process design
- Adhering to standardized work processes

- Promoting effective team functioning
- Encouraging the use of technology
- Creating a learning environment

Prevention by the Physician or Nurse

Although pharmacists are primarily responsible for providing medications, other health care professionals, including physicians and nurses, have a role to play in preventing medication incidents. Appendix B provides links to recommendations for prescription writing, verbal orders, and medication administration made by NCC/MERP and IHI.[13,24] The American Society of Health-System Pharmacists (ASHP) also provides guidelines for nurses and physicians to prevent medication errors in hospitals.[25] Some of these recommendations are summarized below.

Preventive Strategies Regarding Prescribing

Physicians, nurses, and others (including pharmacists) who have authority for prescribing medications should:

- Gather a complete patient history and review the patient's history before prescribing.
- Use preprinted prescription forms or send prescriptions electronically when possible.
- Use computer assistance such as computerized order entry (CPOE) or other management systems.
- Print (instead of writing) words on the prescription.
- Write complete orders, including all pertinent information about the drug (e.g., dosage form, dosage) and patient (e.g., age, weight, diagnosis or purpose of medication) and desired therapeutic outcome.
- Highlight or circle dosages.
- Avoid verbal orders except for emergencies and never for chemotherapy.
- Allow only a physician or properly trained nurse to give oral prescriptions by phone and only pharmacists to receive them.
- If a verbal order is necessary, spell out the drug and patient names, enunciate clearly, and clarify confusing letters (e.g., "S as in Sam"); provide complete information; have the pharmacist read back the order; and document the order in writing.
- Ensure the patient is aware of the purpose of medications being prescribed and discuss any changes to previous orders.
- Contact the pharmacist when prescribing to confirm drug name, dosage, etc., if not 100% certain of the medication information.
- Never use abbreviations for drug names.
- Use only approved Latin abbreviations (e.g., do not use "IN" for "intranasal," as it is mistaken for "IM" or "IV"; rather write out the word "intranasal").
- Use only the metric system except for medications that use standard units, such as insulin.

- Use oral medications where possible.
- Avoid confusing instructions and make sure "hold" orders are clear.

Regarding Administration

Personnel involved in administering medications to patients should:

- Be familiar with indication, precautions and contraindications; expected outcome of use; potential adverse reactions and actions to take if they occur; storage.
- Have access to patient information, including medical history, allergies, diagnosis, current medications, and treatment plan.
- Prior to administration, double-check that it is the right medication, right dose, right person, right route, right dosage form, right time, and right documentation.
- Clarify orders before administration if they are incomplete, illegible, require large volumes or number of dosage forms (e.g., more than two capsules or ampules) or of any concern.
- Do not remove medication from packaging or labeling until immediately before administration.
- Report missing medication and never "borrow" from another patient's supply.
- Listen, ask questions, and double-check orders when a patient objects or questions the administration of medication.
- Understand the proper use of administration devices.

Prevention by the Pharmacy Technician

As part of the pharmacy team, pharmacy technicians also have a role to play in preventing medication incidents, particularly in relation to dispensing errors. Recommendations have been made by NCC-MERP to prevent medication errors (see Appendix B). Some of these and others are summarized here[24,26]:

- Be adequately trained to be familiar with drug names and to understand the importance of accuracy.
- Minimize distractions (e.g., do not engage in non-work-related conversation while filling prescriptions).
- Take responsibility for certain job functions (i.e., answering the phone), so the that pharmacist can focus on providing the medication to the patient.
- Double-check orders (i.e., tech-check-tech [if allowed by state law] pharmacist-check-tech, tech-check-pharmacist).
- Ensure that a pharmacist reviews medication orders and prescriptions prior to dispensing.
- Read labels at least three times (e.g., when selecting the product, when packaging the product, and when returning the product to the shelf).
- Do not override computer alerts when entering prescriptions, particularly those involving drug interactions or potential allergies.

- Triple-check replenishment of regular medication stock or automated dispensing machines/cabinets.
- Highlight strengths and dosage forms (e.g., gel, cream) on manufacturer's drug labeling when there are multiple strengths or dosage forms available.
- Check every number in drug identification numbers, such as the National Drug Code (NDC) numbers.
- Double-check pediatric age and dosage (e.g., clarify if 1 mL or 1 TSP) and input information using metric (e.g., 5 mL rather than 1 TSP).
- Clarify the patient's name and address and ensure complete patient data when receiving a prescription from a patient, inputting the prescriptions in the computer, and prior to handing out a prescription.
- Ensure that a pharmacist is involved in handing out prescription (and counseling) and answering any questions about prescription or nonprescription medications.
- Maintain good housekeeping in the dispensing area and utilize organizational aids (e.g., baskets to keep one patient's prescriptions together, baskets to keep medications for reshelving, and reshelving promptly).
- Keep personal track of medication incidents or errors that you are involved in individually and review these regularly to identify common problems and areas for improvement.
- Report any incidents that occur and participate in investigations.

Prevention by the Patient or Caregiver

It should not be forgotten that patients are also part of the patient care team and that they too have a role in preventing medication incidents. Many organizations have addressed this issue and made recommendations for patients, including the ASHP and the FDA's Center for Drug Evaluation and Research (FDA-CDER).[25,27] Specific recommendations have been made regarding seniors, children, traveling with medications, and emergency preparedness.[25,27] Health care providers can inform patients about these at the time of medication provision. Offering each patient a pamphlet about medication safety would be a good way of doing this, and such pamphlets should be included in public education programs and programs in schools. These involve knowledge about medication and safe handling.

Knowledge about Medication

Patients and caregivers should inform themselves in regard to the following:

- Ask the doctor about the prescriptions he or she is prescribing and whether any changes have been made.
- Always speak directly to the pharmacist even if medications are being delivered to your home.
- Ask the pharmacist the name and purpose of the medication, side effects to watch out for, precautions, nonprescription drug interactions, etc., and make sure you understand all this.

- Keep a complete, up-to-date history of medications and health conditions to share with all health care providers.
- Tell all health care providers about anything that affects your ability to take medications, such as difficulty remembering, or if you are pregnant or might become pregnant or are nursing a baby.
- Ask about possible interactions with current medication before taking any new medication, including dietary supplements or herbal medications.
- Ask for a reasonable explanation if a medication incident occurs and seek assurances that the incident will be thoroughly investigated.

Handling Medications

- Verify medications by sight before leaving the pharmacy.
- Read the label and follow directions.
- Do not change how a medication is used without consulting a health professional.
- Keep medications in original labeled containers.
- Use child-resistant closures on medicines.
- Dispose of medications through the pharmacy or another safe disposal arrangement for hazardous materials.

Prevention by the Pharmacist

Many recommendations have been made regarding the role of the pharmacist in preventing medication incidents by such organizations as ASHP and Canadian Society of Health-System Pharmacists (CSHP).[25,28] The Institute for Safe Medication Practices continually makes recommendations on specific issues identified through incident reports and distributes these via a newsletter, the *ISMP Medication Safety Alert*, to institutional and ambulatory pharmacies. Recommendations have been made in regard to pharmacists' work environments, knowledge and professional practices, dispensing practices, and communication.

The Pharmacists' Work Environment

Where possible, pharmacists should modify their working conditions in regard to the following:

- Arrange shifts and workload appropriately so that shifts are of reasonable length with sufficient staffing to ensure steady and reasonable workload i.e. not too busy but not too slow.[29]
- Reduce distractions in the work area including limiting non-work-related conversation and noise of cash registers, telephones, and printers.
- Attend to work flow and organization so that tasks from receiving prescription to delivery to patient are clearly defined and work flows smoothly with minimum of confusion.

Knowledge and Professional Practices

Pharmacists can use their pharmacy knowledge and good practices to prevent medication incidents by observing the following strategies:

- Use technology to help reduce errors and have proper training to use it.
- Keep up to date with current issues, new drugs and dosing information.
- Do not give advice outside your area of expertise.
- Document all activities, particularly clarification of orders with other health care professionals and discussions with patients.
- Keep personal track of errors and near misses that you are involved in. See Chapter 9 for a personal tracking form.[31]
- Report incidents so that others become aware and can learn from the experience and that preventive measures can be put in place.
- Participate in pharmacy and pharmacist assessments for safe medication practices and work toward developing a patient safety plan.
- Participate in continuous quality improvement (CQI), conducting a risk analysis of your practice site for new products or procedures and a root cause analysis when incidents occur (discussed in Chapter 9).

Dispensing Practices

When they are involved in dispensing prescriptions, pharmacists should observe the following preventive strategies:

- Gather a complete patient history and review the patient's history before dispensing or giving advice.
- Never override or circumvent forcing functions or alerts without a good reason, which is documented.
- Have an independent double-check of orders and completed prescriptions.
- Ensure that medications are delivered to patient, caregiver, or patient-care areas in a safe and timely manner and administered and stored appropriately.
- Obtain any missing or unclear information and never make assumptions or guess the intent of confusing medication orders.
- Never use and never allow others to use the following statements, as suggested by ISMP, to dissuade you from following-up on an issue[30]:
  - "That is what the doctor ordered."
  - "The patient (or caregiver) says that's how they take it at home."
  - "This is a special case."
  - "The dose is from the patient's old chart."
  - "We always give it that way."
  - "I was told to order it that way."

Communication

The following strategies involving communication issues can also help the pharmacist to prevent medication incidents:

- Document all activities, particularly clarification of orders with other health care professionals, and discussions with patients.
- Show the patient his or her medication when counseling.
- Speak directly to the patient if appropriate (rather than a caregiver) whenever possible.
- Maintain good patient and professional relations to improve communication and the gathering of important information.

SUMMARY

If pharmacists and health care organizations where pharmacists practice engage in the risk management and preventive strategies described in this chapter, it is hoped that medication incidents will never occur. Unfortunately, as a result of both immediate and root causes, there are many opportunities for error. Specific strategies have been devised to further avert various types of medication incidents and to address their causes throughout the system and in the pharmacy. These are described in detail in the following four chapters.

Reflective Questions

1. List the elements of risk management for medication incidents.
2. Go to two of the Web sites in Appendix B and note the recommendations made regarding patient safety or the prevention of medication incidents. Discuss the potential value for these Web sites.
3. Review the preventive strategies for organizations, pharmacies, pharmacists, and pharmacy technicians. Discuss what is needed in your own practice (or a typical pharmacy you are familiar with) and the organization of which it is a part (e.g., pharmacy chain) to put these strategies in place.

REFERENCES

1. World Health Organizaiton. Committee of Experts on Management of Safety and Quality in Health Care. Expert Group on Safe Medication Practices. Glossary of terms related to patient and medication safety. Geneva: Council of Europe, World Health Organization, October 2005. Available at: www.who.int/patientsafety/highlights/COE_patient_and_medication_safety_gl.pdf. Accessed July 6, 2006.
2. Joint Commission on Accreditation of Healthcare Organizations (JCAHO). Sentinel Event Glossary of Terms. Available at: www.jointcommission.org/SentinelEvents/se_glossary.htm. Accessed July 7, 2006.
3. Reason J. Human error: models and management. *BMJ.* 2000;320:768–770.
4. Ackroyd-Stolarz S, Hartnell N, MacKinnon N. Approaches to improving the safety of the medication use system. *Healthc Q.* 2005;8(Oct):59–64.

5. Gardner JP, Baker G, Norton P, et al. Governments and patient safety in Australia, the United Kingdom and the United States: a review of policies, institutional and funding frameworks, and current initiatives: final report. Advisory Committee on Health Services Working Group on Quality of Health Care Services, Health Canada, 2002. Available at: www.hc-sc.gc.ca/hcs-sss/pubs/care-soins/2002-gov-patient-securit/index_e.html/. Accessed September 2006.

6. Altman D, Clancy C, Blendon R. Improving patient safety—five years after the IOM report. N Engl J Med. 2004;351(20):2041–2043.

7. Last week was National Patient Safety Week—and what a week it was! ISMP Safety Alert. 2003. March 20. Available at: www.ismp.org/Newsletters/acutecare/articles/20030320.asp. Accessed September 2006.

8. ISMP Responds to new patient safety legislation, Institute for Safe Medication Practices media release, August 3, 2005. Available at: www.ismp.org/pressroom/PR20050803.pdf. Accessed September 2006.

9. Jackson M, Reines W. A systematic approach to preventing medication errors. US Pharm. June 2003. Available at: www.uspharmacist.com/oldformat.asp?url_ce/2790/default.htm. Accessed September 2006.

10. California Board of Pharmacy. California Code of Regulations Add Title 16 CCR, Division 17. Available at: www.pharmacy.ca.gov/laws-regs/1711.pdf. Accessed September 2006.

11. ISMP comments on IOM report, Preventing Medication Errors. ISMP Med Safety Alert. Community/Ambulatory Care Edition. 2006;5(8):1–2.

12. National Steering Committee on Patient Safety. Building a safer system—a national integrated strategy for improving patient safety in Canadian health care. September 2002. Available at: http://rcpsc.medical.org/publications/building_a_safer_e.pdf/. Accessed July 2006.

13. Institute for Healthcare Improvement. Changes in medication systems. Available at: www.ihi.org/IHI/Topics/PatientSafety/MedicationSystems/Changes/. Accessed September 2006.

14. Fleming M. Patient safety culture measurement and improvement: a "how to" guide. Healthc Q. 2005;8(Oct):14–19.

15. Singer SJ, Gaba DM, Geppert AD, et al. The culture of safety: results of an organization wide survey in 15 California hospitals. Q Saf Healthc. 2003;12:112–118.

16. Ginsburg L, Norton P, Casebeer A, et al. An educational intervention to enhance nurse leaders' perceptions of patient safety culture. Health Serv Res, 2005;4: 997–1020. Available at: www.findarticles.com/p/articles/mi_m4149/ai_n15338153. Accessed September 2006.

17. Measuring medication safety: What works? What doesn't? ISMP Med Safety Alert, 1999. Available at: www.ismp.org/Newsletters/acutecare/articles/199990811_2.asp. Accessed September 2006.

18. ISMP's List of High Alert Medications. December 2003. Available at: www.ismp.org/Newsletters/acutecare/articles/20031201.asp?ptr=y. Accessed September 2006.

19. Massachusetts Hospital Association. MHA best practice recommendations to reduce medication errors. Executive summary. Burlington, MA: Massachusetts Coalition for the Prevention of Medical Errors. Massachusetts Hospital Association, 1999. Available at: www.macoalition.org/document/Best_Practices_Medication_Errors.pdf/. Accessed September 2006.

20. Kohn LT, Corrigan JM, Donaldson M, et al, eds. To Err is Human: Building a Safer Health System. Washington, DC: National Academy Press, Institute of Medicine, 1999. Available at: www.nap.edu/html/to_err_is_human. Accessed May 2, 2004.

21. Institute for Safe Medication Practices. Frequently asked questions. Available at: www.ismp.org/faq.asp/. Accessed July 7, 2006.
22. ISPM. Building a case for medication reconciliation. *ISMP Med Saf Alert*, 2005; 10(8). Available at: www.medscape.com/viewarticle/505420/. Accessed September 2005.
23. The Joint Commission. Using medication reconciliatin to prevent errors. *Sentinel Event Alert*. 2006;35. Available at: www.jointcommission.org/SentinelEvents/SentinelEventAlert/sea_35.htm. Accessed September 2007.
24. National Coordinating Council on Medication Error Reporting and Prevention. Council Recommendations. Available at: www.nccmerp.org/councilRecs.html. Accessed September 2006.
25. American Society of Hospital Pharmacists. ASHP guidelines on preventing medication errors in hospitals. *Am J Hosp Pharm*. 1993;50:305–314. Available at: www.ashp.org/s_ashp/bin.asp?CID=6&DID=5426&DOC=FILE.PDF. Accessed September 2007.
26. 7 ways to prevent medication errors. Tech Talk. *Pharm Pract*. 2002;18(1):1.
27. U.S. Food and Drug Administration. Center for Drug Evaluation and Research (CDER). Think it through: a guide to managing the benefits and risks of medicines. Consumer Information. Available at: www.fda.gov/cder/consumerinfo/think.htm/. Accessed September 2006.
28. Canadian Society of Hospital Pharmacists. Impact of hospital pharmacists on patient safety. Background paper. December, 2003. Available at: www.cshp.ca/dms/dmsView/1_safety.pdf. Accessed September 2006.
29. Grasha A. Misconceptions about pharmacy workload. *CPJ*. 2001;134(3):26–35.
30. ISPM. Patient safety is all about taking that extra step. *ISMP Med Saf Alert*, July 11, 2001. Available at: www.ismp.org/MSAarticles/extrastep.html. Accessed July 7, 2004.
31. Grasha A. Using self-monitoring, personal feedback and goal setting to reduce error. *Qual Assur Health Notes*. 2002;1(6):19–24. Available at: http://pharmacy.ucsf.edu/ce/qa/qa.pdf. Accessed September 2006.

Chapter 4

Common Causes of Medication Incidents and Preventive Strategies

Objectives

After completing this chapter, the reader will be able to:

- Recognize various types of medication incidents frequently seen in pharmacy practice
- Identify similar situations in your practice that could lead to medication incidents
- Identify contributory factors and preventive strategies for common causes of medication incidents
- Apply the knowledge gained to current practice with a view to the prevention of future incidents

Research shows that the causes of medication errors are complex. Each incident, when examined closely, is made up of many contributory factors. The causes of a variety of medication incidents are here examined in more detail, using a case study approach to analyze the factors that play a role in an incident. Pharmacists and pharmacy technicians are in a key position in the medication process to offer insight into what went wrong—in an atmosphere that does not assign blame. A number of preventive strategies that may be used to decrease errors are discussed throughout this chapter.

The cornerstone of error prevention is effective communication. When it works well, patients receive high-quality care. However, failed communication can lead to medication errors, with sometimes tragic consequences. Some examples of communication errors that have led to medication incidents include illegible handwriting, poor verbal communication, fax errors, sound-alike and look-alike drug names, missing information, and inappropriate use of symbols and abbreviations.

ILLEGIBLE HANDWRITING

Poor handwriting on prescriptions is a widely recognized cause of medication incidents. A January 2003 report on incidents at all hospitals in Winnipeg, Manitoba, ranks illegible handwriting as the top cause of incidents.[1] Misunderstanding of the intended drug, dosage, route of administration, or frequency can result from illegible prescriptions. Workflow can be interrupted when pharmacy staff attempt the time-consuming task of clarifying illegible handwriting. As a result, patient care can be delayed, as Cases 4.1 and 4.2 illustrate.

Case 4.1

The handwritten prescription shown here, for an 80-year-old patient, was interpreted and dispensed as ferrous sulfate 300 mg to be taken once daily. While counseling on the use of ferrous sulfate, the pharmacist was interrupted by the patient, who indicated that the medication should be for her leg cramps. On contacting the physician, it was confirmed that he intended to prescribe quinine sulfate 300 mg.

Possible Contributory Factors

- Poor physician handwriting.
- "Ferrous sulfate" and "quinine sulfate" can look alike when poorly written.
- Both drugs are available in the 300-mg strength and can be taken once daily.

Case 4.2

A 60-year-old patient took the prescription shown here to his local pharmacy for filling. In error, the pharmacy technician interpreted and entered the prescription into the computer as Hytrin 10 mg, whereas the physician had intended to prescribe Lipitor 10 mg. Upon checking the prescription, the pharmacist did not detect the error. A few hours later, the patient returned to pick up the medication. When the pharmacist tried to provide patient counseling, the patient indicated that he had been taking the medication for some time and, therefore, did not require any further information. The patient, therefore, left the pharmacy with the incorrect medication. Fortunately, the patient called the pharmacy before taking any of the tablets when he noticed that they did not look the same as his usual pills.

Possible Contributory Factors

- Poor physician handwriting.
- Both drugs have the same dosage form, strength, and route of administration.
- The patient's medication history was not checked by the pharmacist.
- The pharmacist's attempt to provide counseling failed.
- The indication for use was missing from the written prescription.

Preventive Strategies for Illegible Prescriptions

- Contact the prescriber to clarify any ambiguous prescriptions.
- Use the patient's medication history as a tool to confirm or clarify unclear prescriptions.
- Patient counseling at the time of dispensing is a key step in preventing medication errors. At a minimum, the patient should be asked, "What were you told this medication is for?" "How were you told to take this medication?" and "What were you told to expect from this medication?"
- If appropriate, meet with individual prescribers to discuss the serious nature of this issue and the impact on patient outcomes.
- Whenever possible, the person entering the prescription into the computer should not be the same person who is checking the prescription.
- While counseling the patient, consider opening the vial to give you and the patient both a chance to confirm the contents before the patient leaves the pharmacy.
- With the availability of computerized technology—which can produce clear, legible, and complete prescriptions—handwritten prescriptions should be a thing of the past. Physicians and other prescribers should be encouraged to use available computerized technology in prescribing medications. With the use of computerized physician order entry (CPOE), the prescriber enters the order directly into a computer or handheld device. The system can then guide him or her through the medication ordering process. CPOE systems can suggest the drug of choice, provide dosage suggestions and dosing intervals, and can alert the prescriber to drug allergy, contraindications and drug–drug interactions. All stakeholders—including governments, pharmacy organizations, physician organizations, pharmacists, pharmacy technicians, physicians, and the public—must advocate for the reduction and eventual discontinuation of handwritten prescriptions.

LOOK-ALIKE/SOUND-ALIKE MEDICATIONS

The existence of a large number of look-alike/sound-alike drug names can also be a factor in the misinterpretation of the prescriber's intent. The potential for error is compounded when the two look-alike/sound-alike products are available in the same strength (e.g., Ceftin 250 mg and Cefzil 250 mg) or with the same directions (twice daily), dosage form (oral tablets), and similar clinical indications (antibiotic).

Problems can occur not only because the drug names look alike but also because of similar product packaging. This problem is magnified if products from the same drug company are stocked next to each other on the dispensary shelf.

Complete information on a prescription is essential to achieving positive outcomes. Each jurisdiction has legislation that details the requirements for a complete prescription, and the lack of any aspect of the required information may increase the risk of medication incidents. An extremely important piece of information that is not mandatory and, therefore, often missing is the indication for use or purpose of the medication. The indication for use provides the pharmacist and the pharmacy technician with an additional tool to clarify ambiguous prescriptions and confirm that the physician's intent has been correctly interpreted. This is particularly useful in preventing medication errors associated with look-alike/sound-alike drug names (e.g., hydroxyzine and hydralazine). In some cases, drugs that are not usually considered look-alike may actually look the same when written.

In 1997, the Motherisk program in Canada (an evidence-based source of information about the safety or risk of drugs during pregnancy and lactation) became aware of 10 confirmed cases of dispensing errors in which pregnant women received Dicetel instead of Diclectin. The duration of exposure varied from a day to a month before the error was detected. All 10 women took part in a follow-up interview to determine the outcomes of their pregnancies. Nine delivered healthy babies and the tenth experienced a spontaneous abortion a week following the ingestion of Dicetel.[2]

Medication errors involving the sound-alike and look-alike drug pair Amaryl (glimepiride) and Reminyl (galantamine) have occurred in Canada and in the United States. In an effort to prevent future dispensing errors, the manufacturer of Reminyl announced that the brand name Reminyl will be changed to Razadyne in the United States.[3] The manufacturers of Reminyl must be congratulated for taking this key step to support patient safety. However, it is puzzling that the change in name from Reminyl to Razadyne is being implemented only in the United States when the potential for error also exists in Canada.

Similarly, after the launch of Losec (omeprazole), this drug was often confused with Lasix (furosemide).[4] A number of medication errors were reported as a result. The name "Losec" was, therefore, changed to "Prilosec" in the United States. Yet, Losec remains the brand name in Canada, where the potential for a medication mixup and possible patient harm still exists.

Steps taken by pharmaceutical manufacturers to enhance patient safety must extend beyond the borders of the United States. Actions such as a change in drug name should occur in all countries in which the potential for a mixup exists. Patient safety is a global issue.

Cases 4.3 and 4.4 illustrate the potential for error with look-alike/sound-alike medications.

Case 4.3

Amiloride tabs
Sig: i qam
Dispense: 30

Upon entering this prescription into the computer, the pharmacy technician selected Apo-amilzide (amiloride/hydrochlorothiazide) tablets instead of the potassium-sparing diuretic amiloride (Midamor), as the prescription indicated. The pharmacist checked the prescription but did not detect the computer entry error. When the patient received the medication, the pharmacist's counseling of the patient included discussion of the indication for use (diuretic) and confirmed the directions (once daily in the morning). The patient left the pharmacy and began to take the incorrect medication according to the directions confirmed with the pharmacist.

One month later, the patient called the pharmacy to request a refill of his medication. The pharmacist then contacted the physician for an authorization to refill the Apo-amilzide, and the error was discovered. Fortunately the patient did not suffer any long-term effects. However, the pharmacist–physician relationship was then strained and a lack of trust developed on the part of the patient.

Possible Contributory Factors

- The drugs have look-alike names.
- Both drugs have the same dosage form and directions for use as well as similar indications.
- The physician did not indicate the strength of the medication.

Case 4.4

A 47-year-old female patient presented the prescription shown here for processing. The pharmacy technician entered the prescription into the computer as metoprolol 100 mg to be taken three times daily. The pharmacist checked the prescription but did not detect the computer entry error.

On counseling the patient, the pharmacist explained that the tablets should be taken on a regular basis to reduce her blood pressure. The patient responded that the tablets were not intended to reduce blood pressure. A closer look at the written prescription revealed that the prescription was written for misoprostol 100 μg. The pharmacist apologized for the error and made the correction.

Possible Contributory Factors

- The words "metoprolol" and "misoprostol" can look alike when poorly written.
- The pharmacist read 100 mg instead of 100 μg.
- The pharmacist did not consider the appropriateness of the dosing interval and duration of therapy for metoprolol.
- The pharmacist read the computer-generated hard copy before reading the actual written prescription. As a result, the pharmacist was misled by the technician's misinterpretation of the prescriber's intent and was likely biased in arriving at his own interpretation of the prescription.
- Metoprolol is prescribed more often than misoprostol. Therefore, both the pharmacy technician and the pharmacist likely "saw" what was most familiar. This is often referred to as confirmation bias.

Preventive Strategies for Look-Alike/ Sound-Alike Medications

- Always contact the prescriber to clarify an ambiguous prescription.
- Whenever possible, the pharmacist checking the prescription should NOT be the same individual who entered the prescription in the computer.
- Ensure that all staff are aware of problematic look-alike/sound-alike drug names often involved in medication errors (see Table 4.1). An extensive list may be found at www.usp.org/pdf/EN/patientSafety/qr792004-04-01.pdf.
- Place cautionary labels/stickers on look-alike/sound-alike drugs to alert pharmacy staff of the potential for error (see Fig. 4.1).
- Add auxiliary labels to the manufacturer's label to visually differentiate two drugs with similar names (See Fig. 4.2).
- Physically separate look-alike/sound-alike drugs from each other on the pharmacy shelf.
- Consider an alternative to shelving products according to alphabetical classification by product name or manufacturer name. With the use of "prescription mapping" software, products are stored based on frequency of use.[5] As a result, look-alike and sound-alike drugs are not stored next to each other.
- Suggest to your software vendor that alert flags be added to the drug files of look-alike/sound-alike drugs (e.g., flashing screen). As an interim step, a note may be added to the drug file.
- In filling prescriptions, use the original written prescription to select the product from the shelf. Then compare the National Drug Code (United States) or the Drug Identification Number (Canada) of the selected product with the computer-generated hard copy to confirm accuracy.
- Encourage prescribers to include the indication for use on prescriptions. This will make it easier to interpret the prescriber's intent correctly, as look-alike/sound-alike drugs usually have different indications.

TABLE 4.1
Look-Alike/Sound-Alike Medications

Celebrex	Cerebyx
	Celexa
Ceftin	Cefzil
Hycomine	Hycodan
Inderal	Isordil
	Toradol
	Adderall
	Imdur
	Imuran
Lamisil	Lomotil
	Lamictal
Percodan	Percocet
Tobrex	Tobradex
Trusopt	Cosopt
Xanax	Zantac
Xenical	Xeloda
	Senokot
Ampicillin	Amoxicillin
	Aminophylline
Azithromycin	Erythromycin
Chlorpromazine	Chlorpropamide
	Clomipramine
	Prochlorperazine
	Promethazine
	Clomiphene
Dimenhydrinate	Diphenhydramine
Enalapril	Ramipril

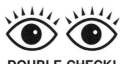

DOUBLE-CHECK!

LOOK-ALIKE DRUGS

FIGURE 4.1 Sample cautionary sticker.

| HydrALAzine | | hydrOXYzine |

FIGURE 4.2 Sample auxiliary labels.

- In dispensing a specific drug, consider all aspects of the prescription for appropriateness. Factors to be considered include patient parameters, the dose, dosing interval, duration of therapy, etc.
- Provide effective patient counseling and discuss the purpose of the medication. Encourage patients to ask questions, particularly when something seems different or unusual.
- Check the patient's medication history to help determine the prescriber's intent.
- Educate patients on what to expect in taking a medication and advise them to report any unexpected side effects.
- Pharmaceutical manufacturers must perform adequate failure analysis of proposed trademarks to identify potential problems. This analysis should occur during both the prelaunch and postmarketing phases.

VERBAL PRESCRIPTIONS

There is a greater risk of error in receiving verbal prescriptions as compared with written or electronic prescriptions. Verbally communicated prescriptions are often misheard, misinterpreted, or mistranscribed. Other factors contributing to failed verbal communication include poor pronunciation by the prescriber, unclear speech as a result of an accent, sound-alike brand names or generic names, and hearing deficiencies on the part of the receiver. In addition, office staff not familiar with a specific drug may mispronounce or misspell its name.

Background noise, interruptions and the use of unfamiliar terminology can compound the problem. In addition, once received, the verbal instructions must be transcribed to written prescriptions. The possibility of a transcription error is, therefore, introduced. There is an even greater risk of error when a nurse or secretary receives a verbal instruction from a prescriber and subsequently telephones the prescription into the pharmacy.

Consider the following case of a verbal prescription, which could have had significant consequences.

Case 4.5

A physician telephoned a community pharmacy to give a verbal prescription for what the pharmacist heard as 60 Senokot tablets, to be taken as directed. The prescription was then filled and placed in a drawer for pickup.

Later that day, the patient arrived to pick up her prescription. The pharmacist began to provide counseling on the use of Senokot tablets and was interrupted by the patient, who said, "There must be a mistake; my doctor ordered Xenical." Upon further investigation, it was found that the pharmacist had misheard the physician.

Possible Contributory Factors

- The prescriber spoke with an accent. As a result, Xenical sounded like Senokot.

- Physicians often prescribe both Senokot and Xenical without indicating a specific strength. An indication of the strength in this instance could have been useful in differentiating between the two drugs.

- No specific directions were given. Vague directions such as "take as directed" reduce the likelihood of detecting a potential error before a drug reaches the patient.

- Xenical was newly introduced into the market. The pharmacist, therefore, heard what he was most familiar with (i.e., Senekot).

- No indication for the prescription was given.

Preventive Strategies for Verbal Prescriptions

- Discourage the use of verbal prescriptions except in emergencies.
- Receive verbal prescriptions in an area of the pharmacy where noise and other distractions are minimized.
- Always repeat the prescription, as understood by you, to the prescriber to verify accuracy. Whenever possible, repeat both the brand and generic names.
- Repeat numbers in the teens the way pilots state numbers. For example, "one-five" milligrams instead of "fifteen" milligrams.
- If the prescriber is rushed and unable to wait while you repeat the prescription, fax a written record of the prescription to the prescriber's office for verification before dispensing.
- If possible, find out the purpose of the medication.
- Write the prescription as understood directly onto a prescription pad. Avoid having to rewrite the prescription from a scrap of paper, as this can introduce the possibility of a transcription error.
- Record the name of the caller, the date, and time the prescription was received.
- Ensure that effective patient counseling takes place with all prescriptions; this should include a discussion of the purpose of the medication.
- Supplement verbal counseling with written information at the time of counseling and review it with the patient.

FAXED PRESCRIPTIONS

Faxed prescriptions are appropriate in some instances where permitted by law, particularly when a written prescription is required. They can avoid some of the inherent difficulties of verbal orders but retain the characteristics of written orders. Faxed prescriptions can be an effective tool for reducing the number of phone calls to the pharmacy and thus help to decrease noise, distraction, and interruptions. However, the distortion that may occur on faxed prescriptions can lead to misinterpretation, as seen in Case 4.6.

Case 4.6

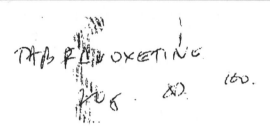

The prescription shown here was faxed to a community pharmacy for filling. The prescription was interpreted and processed as paroxetine 20 mg once daily. The pharmacist began to counsel the patient on paroxetine. However, the patient indicated that he had expected a refill of the Prozac (fluoxetine) capsules he was currently taking. Upon contacting the physician's office for verification, the pharmacist learned that the prescriber had intended to prescribe fluoxetine and not paroxetine.

Possible Contributory Factors

- Poor quality of fax.
- Poorly written prescription.
- Fluoxetine and paroxetine can look alike when poorly written.
- Both drugs are available in 20-mg oral dosage forms.
- Both drugs are usually taken once daily.
- The patient was new to the pharmacy; therefore, a medication history was not readily available.

Preventive Strategies for Faxed Prescriptions

- Examine each fax carefully. Look for lines, streaks, and other marks that may be misinterpreted.
- If unsure of the prescriber's intent, contact him or her for clarification.
- Ensure routine maintenance of fax machines.
- Whenever possible, compare the faxed order with the written order.

MISSING INFORMATION

Although a prescription may be written with good penmanship, there may still be the potential for misinterpretation of the physician's intention if the order is missing information such as dosage form, indication, or route of administration. Assumptions may be made which can lead to the incorrect medication being dispensed, as Cases 4.7 and 4.8 illustrate.

Case 4.7

A patient presented the following prescription to a pharmacy technician for filling.

Garamycin Oint
Sig: Apply tid
Dispense: 1 tube

The technician entered the prescription into the computer as Garamycin Topical Ointment. On checking the prescription, the pharmacist also assumed that the physician intended to prescribe the topical ointment. As a result, one 15-g tube of Garamycin Topical Ointment was dispensed. While counseling the patient on the use of the ointment, the patient interrupted the pharmacist, saying "I thought this was for my eyes!" On contacting the physician, it was confirmed that he had intended to prescribe Garamycin Ophthalmic Ointment.

Case 4.8

The prescription shown here, which was written for a 50-year-old patient, was taken to a community pharmacy for processing. The technician interpreted and entered the prescription into the computer as 5 g MetroGel (metronidazole 0.75%), to be applied topically once daily for 5 days. Therefore, 5 g of Metrogel was weighed and put into a jar. The pharmacist checked the prescription and accepted the technician's interpretation as correct.

A few hours later, the patient returned for the medication. The pharmacist retrieved the jar and began to counsel the patient on the use of the gel topically. The patient appeared puzzled and told the pharmacist that she was sure that the physician had prescribed a vaginal product to be inserted at bedtime for 5 nights.

The pharmacist then rechecked the prescription and realized that the prescriber had written the prescription for metronidazole vaginal gel. The physician intended that the patient insert one applicator (5 g) once daily (at bedtime) for 5 nights.

The pharmacist apologized for the error and provided the correct medication and instructions for use.

Possible Contributory Factors

- There are a number of metronidazole 0.75% products, including MetroGel, MetroCream, MetroLotion, and MetroGel Vaginal (United States)/NidaGel (Canada). Therefore, the prescription as written is incomplete and ambiguous.

- The physician did not include the indication for use, the route of administration, or the specific quantity to be dispensed.
- The pharmacist and pharmacy technician were not aware that 5 g as written on the prescription referred to the quantity of gel per applicator.

Preventive Strategies for Prescriptions with Missing Information

- Always contact the prescriber to clarify incomplete prescriptions where the dosage form or route of administration is missing.
- Do not dispense the medication until the prescriber's intent has been confirmed. If the patient must begin therapy before this occurs, use professional judgment and provide a minimal number of doses.
- Consider the appropriateness of the quantity of drug being dispensed, along with the instructions for use.
- Always check the patient history to identify previous and current medications being taken.
- The patient is often a key source of information. Ask "What were you told the medication is for?" and "How were you told to take it?"

ABBREVIATIONS AND SYMBOLS

The use of Latin abbreviations is common in pharmacy practice. In an effort to save time, abbreviations and symbols are often used by prescribers in writing prescriptions. Although their use may save time and be habitual for prescribers, their misinterpretation has led to numerous medication incidents. A poorly written abbreviation may be misinterpreted for another abbreviation. In addition, a nonstandard abbreviation may be unfamiliar to the pharmacist or technician who is attempting to interpret the prescription. Cases 4.9, 4.10, and 4.11 illustrate the potential for harm.

Case 4.9

Omeprazole 20mg SID

A veterinarian wrote the prescription shown here for animal use. The pharmacy technician processed the prescription as omeprazole 20 mg, with the directions to take one tablet twice daily. Upon checking the prescription, the pharmacist identified the dosage as unusual. The prescriber was contacted and the dosage was confirmed to be one tablet daily. The veterinarian had used the Latin abbreviation s.i.d. (*semel in die*) to mean once daily.[6] Although this is commonly used in veterinary practice, it is unfamiliar to most pharmacists and pharmacy technicians.

Case 4.10

A physician prescribed atenolol 50-mg tablets to be taken once daily. The pharmacy technician entered the directions for use into the computer as "T 1 TAB OD" which was translated as "Take one tablet in the right eye." Upon checking the prescription, the pharmacist did not detect the error. The patient followed the instructions given verbally and correctly took one tablet orally once daily. However, a few days later the patient read the prescription label and returned to the pharmacy for an explanation. Although there was no patient harm, the pharmacist's credibility was probably affected.

Case 4.11

A 70-year-old patient presented the following prescription to her local community pharmacy for filling:

Zocor 20 mg
Sig: i tab daily cc
Dispense: 30

The prescription was processed with the label instructions to "Take one tablet daily with meals." The correct medication was dispensed to the patient. On returning home, the patient began to take one tablet with *each* meal.

Approximately 10 days later, the patient returned to the pharmacy for a refill of her medication. Upon questioning the patient regarding the need for an early refill, the pharmacist discovered that the patient had been taking one tablet three times daily instead of once daily as prescribed. Fortunately no ill effects were observed.

Possible Contributory Factors

- Upon entering the prescription into the computer, the technician keyed in the abbreviation "cc" which was translated to "with meals." The technician was not given the option to select "with meals" or "with a meal."
- There was a possible communication barrier, since the patient's mother tongue was not the same as the pharmacist's.
- The pharmacist did not confirm that the patient understood the instructions for taking the medication.

Preventive Strategies for Abbreviations and Symbols

- Contact your software vendor, if necessary, to ensure that abbreviations and codes are translated appropriately and accurately.
- Remind all computer entry technicians to check the translation of all abbreviations before printing a prescription label. Consider whether the patient would correctly interpret the instructions for taking the medication. In Case

4.11, the instructions for use could have been printed as, "Take one tablet *once* daily with *a* meal." Additional written information might also have been given to highlight the evening meal only.

- Encourage prescribers to avoid abbreviations that could be misinterpreted. The complete instructions should be written.
- Always contact the prescriber to clarify potentially confusing or ambiguous abbreviations.
- The technician who prepares and labels the medication should also check the printed label to identify possible computer entry errors.
- During patient counseling, the printed prescription label should also be checked for accuracy.
- Whenever possible, contact the prescriber to clarify ambiguous instructions such as "Take as directed" or "Use as before." In many instances, the patient cannot recall the verbal instructions given by the prescriber. In addition, "Use *as* before" has been erroneously translated to "Use *in the left ear* before."
- Educate all pharmacy staff about problematic abbreviations that may lead to patient harm (see Tables 4.2, 4.3, and 4.4). A more extensive list can be accessed at www.ismp.org/pdf/errorprone.pdf.
- Since a large number of errors occur at the point of computer entry, technicians should be trained to become familiar with the dosage regimens of medications being dispensed.
- In counseling patients, always confirm their understanding of the information provided.

TABLE 4.2
Abbreviations for Instructions

Abbreviation	Intended Meaning	Misinterpretation	Preventive Strategy
AU, AS, AD	Aurio uterque (each ear) left ear, right ear	Mistaken for OU (oculo uterque— each eye), left eye, right eye	Write out full intended meaning
BT	Bedtime	Mistaken for "bid" (twice daily)	Use "bedtime"
cc	Cubic centimeters	Misread as "U" (units)	Use "mL"
D/C	Discharge or discontinue	Premature discontinuation of medications if D/C (intended to mean "discharge") has been misinterpreted as "discontinued" when followed by a list of discharge medications	Use "discharge" and "discontinue"
IN	Intranasal	Mistaken as "IM" or "IV"	Use "intranasal"

(continued)

TABLE 4.2
Abbreviations for Instructions (Continued)

Abbreviation	Intended Meaning	Misinterpretation	Preventive Strategyi
μg	Microgram	Mistaken for "mg" when handwritten	Write out full intended meaning or use mcg.
o.d. or OD	Once daily	Misinterpreted as "right eye" (OD–oculus dexter) and administration of oral medication in the eye.	Write out "daily"
OJ	Orange juice	Mistaken as OD or OS (right or left eye); drugs meant to be diluted in orange juice may be given in the eye.	Use "orange juice"
per os	Orally	The "os" can be mistaken for "left eye."	Use "PO," "by mouth," or "orally"
q.d. or QD	Every day	Mistaken as q.i.d., especially if the period after the "q" or the tail of the "q" is misunderstood as an "i"	Write out "daily"
q.o.d. or QOD	Every other day	Misinterpreted as "q.d." (daily) or "q.i.d." (four times daily) if the "o" is poorly written.	Write out intended meaning or use "q other day"
qhs	At bedtime	Mistaken as "qhr" or every hour	Use "at bedtime"
qn	Nightly	Mistaken as "qh" (every hour)	Use "nightly"
q1d	Daily	Mistaken as "q.i.d." (four times daily)	Use "daily"
SC, SQ, sub q	Subcutaneous	SC mistaken as SL (sublingual; SQ mistaken as "5 every"; the "q" in "sub q" has been mistaken as "every" (e.g., a heparin dose ordered "sub q 2 hours before surgery" misunderstood as "every 2 hours before surgery")	Use "subcutaneously"

(continued)

TABLE 4.2
Abbreviations for Instructions (Continued)

Abbreviation	Intended Meaning	Misinterpretation	Preventive Strategyi
ss	Sliding scale (insulin) or ½ (apothecary)	Mistaken as "55"	Write out "sliding scale"; use "one-half" or "½"
HS	Half strength	Misinterpreted as the Latin abbreviation "HS" (hour of sleep).	Write out strength of medication
hs	At bedtime, hours of sleep	Mistaken as half strength	Use "bedtime"
1/d or i/d	One daily	Mistaken as "tid"	Use "1 daily"
TIW or tiw	3 times a week	Mistaken as "3 times a day" or "twice a week"	Use "3 times weekly"
IU	International unit	Mistaken as IV (intravenous) or 10 (ten)	Use "units"
U or u	Unit	Read as zero (0) or a four (4), causing a 10-fold overdose or greater (4U seen as "40" or 4u seen as "44").	Write out "units"

Adapted with permission from ISMP. List of error-prone abbreviations, symbols, and dose designations. *ISMP Med Saf Alert.* 2003;8(24):1–4.

Abbreviated drug names are another source of potential misinterpretation. While it may seem convenient and perhaps time-saving to abbreviate drug names, it may lead to misunderstanding when the pharmacist or technician is unfamiliar with the abbreviation. Table 4.3 illustrates several instances of potential incidents. In all cases, the preventive strategy is to use the full drug name.

TABLE 4.3
Abbreviations of Drug Names

Drug Name	Intended Meaning	Misinterpretation	Preventive Strategy
AZT	Zidovudine (Retrovir)	Azathioprine (Imuran)	Use full drug name
HCl	Hydrochloric acid	Potassium chloride (KCl)	Use full drug name
HCT	Hydrocortisone	Hydrochlorothiazide (HCTZ)	Use full drug name
HCTZ	Hydrochlorothiazide	Hydrocortisone (HCT)	Use full drug name

(continued)

TABLE 4.3
Abbreviations of Drug Names (Continued)

Drug Name	Intended Meaning	Misinterpretation	Preventive Strategy
MgSO₄	Magnesium sulfate	Morphine sulfate (MS)	Use full drug name
MS	Morphine sulfate	Magnesium sulfate	Use full drug name
MTX	Methotrexate	Mitoxantrone	Use full drug name
Nitro drip	Nitroprusside	Nitroglycerin	Use full drug name
Norflox	Norfloxacin (Noroxin)	Norflex (orphenadrine)	Use full drug name
IV Vanc	Intravenous vancomycin	Invanz (ertapenem sodium)	Use full drug name

Adapted with permission from ISMP. List of error-prone abbreviations, symbols, and dose designations. *ISMP Med Saf Alert.* 2003;8(24):1–4.

Table 4.4 outlines several other symbols that may be misinterpreted.

TABLE 4.4
Potentially Confusing Symbols

Symbol	Intended Meaning	Misinterpretation	Preventive Strategy
ʒ	Dram	Symbol for dram mistaken for "3"	Use the metric system
♏	Minim	Symbol for minim mistaken as "mL"	Use the metric system
X3d	For three days	Mistaken as "3 doses"	Use "for three days"
> and <	Greater than and less than	Mistaken as opposite of intended; mistakenly use incorrect symbol; "<10" mistaken as "40"	Use "greater than" or "less than"
/ (slash mark)	Separates two doses or indicates "per"	Mistaken as the number 1 (e.g., "25 units/ 10 units" misread as "25 units and 110 units")	Use "per" rather than a slash mark to separate doses
@	At	Mistaken as "2"	Use "at"
&	And	Mistaken as "2"	Use "and"
+	Plus or and	Mistaken as "4"	Use "and"
°	Hour	Mistaken as a zero (e.g., q2° seen as q20)	Use "hour"

Adapted with permission from ISMP. List of error-prone abbreviations, symbols, and dose designations. *ISMP Med Saf Alert.* 2003;8(24):1–4.

CALCULATION AND DECIMAL POINT ERRORS

Each day pharmacists and technicians are required to perform a number of arithmetic calculations. These may include the following:

- Determining the appropriate dose for an individual based on patient-specific information, such as weight
- Confirming prescribed dosages, especially for the pediatric population
- Calculating the quantity of each component of an extemporaneous mixture
- Converting apothecary measures to the metric system
- Determining the total volume or quantity of a specific medication to be dispensed based on the dosage and duration of therapy

However, miscalculations are a well-recognized cause of medication errors. In a study conducted to determine the factors related to errors in medication prescribing, it was determined that 17.5% of the errors were due to the use of calculations, decimal points, or unit and rate expression factors.[7] Children are particularly at risk. A recent study by Harvard Medical School found that children are three times as likely as adults to receive the wrong dose of a drug.[8] In another study, 82 of 150 teaching hospital doctors were unable to correctly calculate how many milligrams of lignocaine were in a 10-mL ampule of 1% solution.[9]

In many instances, oral liquids are prescribed in milligrams per dose rather than volume. Pharmacists and technicians must, therefore, calculate the volume of product to be administered, thereby increasing the risk of error. Pharmacists and technicians may also be required to convert drug dosages from a percentage or ratio concentration to a mass concentration.

The following is a simple calculation to solve without the use of a calculator. Take 1,000 and add 40 to it. Now add another 1,000. Now add 30. Add another 1,000. Now add 20. Now add another 1,000. Now add 10. What is the total? It is not 5,000. The correct total is 4,100.

Examples of calculation errors commonly seen in practice include these:

- Inappropriate rounding off of numbers. This is particularly problematic if the calculation requires two or more steps as the error is perpetuated.
- Use of the incorrect drug concentration in calculating the prescribed dose.
- Misplaced decimal points, which can lead to a 10-fold or one-tenth dosing error.

In addition, dosages involving decimal points may be inappropriately written by the prescriber, which can lead to misinterpretation of the intended dose. Pharmacists have reported receiving written prescriptions for levothyroxine 0.25 mg instead of the intended 0.025 mg. These types of errors can result in a 10-fold overdose with potentially disastrous consequences. Cases 4.12 and 4.13 illustrate examples of calculation errors and case 4.14 illustrates a decimal point error.

Case 4.12

A 53-year-old patient presented the following prescription for processing:

2% Testosterone in Glaxal Base
Sig: Apply as directed
Dispense: 100 g

The ingredients selected for compounding the extemporaneous mixture were Depo-testosterone cypionate 100 mg/mL and Glaxal Base Cream. A pharmacy technician determined that 2 mL of Depo-testosterone cypionate 100 mg/mL and 98 g of Glaxal Base Cream would be required to complete the mixture. On checking the prescription, the pharmacist did not detect the calculation error. The resulting mixture, given to the patient, contained only 0.2 g testosterone instead of the intended 2 g.

Approximately a month later, the patient requested a refill of her prescription from a second pharmacy. On this occasion, the prescription was compounded as originally intended. On receiving the compounded product, the patient questioned the difference in the appearance and consistency from the original product. The pharmacist then contacted the original pharmacy and the error was detected.

Case 4.13

Tazorac 0.1% cream: Anthelios 60
1:4
Sig: Apply once daily
Dispense: 60 g

This prescription was presented to a community pharmacy for processing. The physician intended that one part of Tazorac 0.1% cream be combined with four parts Anthelios 60 for a total of 60 g. That is, 12 g of Tazorac 0.1% cream was to be combined with 48 g of Anthelios 60. However, the pharmacy technician misinterpreted the Tazorac 0.1% cream content to be one quarter of the total mixture. Therefore, 15 g of Tazorac 0.1% cream was weighed and combined with 45 g of Anthelios 60. As a result, the mixture contained 25% Tazorac 0.1% cream instead of the intended 20%. Upon checking the prescription, the pharmacist detected the error.

Although the risk of patient harm is low in this case, calculation errors can result in patient morbidity and mortality, especially when drugs with a narrow therapeutic index are being dispensed to pediatric patients.

> ## Case 4.14

The prescription shown here was presented to a pharmacy technician for filling. On processing the prescription, the technician failed to see the decimal point and entered the prescription into the computer as morphine 50-mg tablets. Fortunately the pharmacist detected the error on checking the prescription and dispensed morphine 5-mg tablets, as the prescriber had intended.

Possible Contributory Factors

- The prescriber added an unnecessary decimal point and zero following the number 5.
- The decimal point is barely visible and, therefore, easily missed in a busy environment.

Preventive Strategies for Calculation and Decimal Point Errors

- Ensure that all dosage calculations are independently checked by at least two individuals.
- Use a calculator whenever possible.
- For increased accuracy, ensure that the decimal place on the calculator is not set to zero.
- Consider the patient's age, weight, and body system function in calculating dosages.
- Standardize drug concentrations whenever possible.
- Use computer alerts to highlight dosages outside the normal range.
- In using decimals, remember to use leading zeros for numbers less than 1 (0.1 mg instead of .1 mg), *not* trailing zeroes for numbers greater than 1 (1 mg instead of 1.0 mg) (see Table 4.5).

TABLE 4.5
Proper Use of Decimal Points and Zeros

Dose Designation	Intended Meaning	Misinterpretation	Prevention Strategy
Trailing zero after a decimal point. (e.g., 1.0 mg)	1 mg	Mistaken as 10 mg if the decimal point is not seen	Do not use trailing zeros for doses expressed as whole numbers. *(continued)*

TABLE 4.5
Proper Use of Decimal Points and Zeros (Continued)

Dose Designation	Intended Meaning	Misinterpretation	Prevention Strategy
No leading zero before a decimal dose (e.g., .5 mg)	0.5 mg	Mistaken for 5 mg if the decimal point is not seen	Use zero before a decimal point when the dose is less than a whole unit.

Reprinted with permission from ISMP. List of error-prone abbreviations, symbols, and dose designations. *ISMP Med Saf Alert.* 2003;8(24):1–4.

DRUG DEVICE ERRORS

Drug devices can also be a source of medication errors. Between 1987 and March 2003, Health Canada received reports of 425 separate incidents involving infusion pumps. Of the 425 incidents, 23 resulted in death, 135 resulted in injury, and 127 could potentially have led to death or injury.[10]

The July 10, 2003, ISMP (Institute for Safe Medication Practices) Medication Safety Alert highlighted many of the problems associated with the use of patient-controlled analgesia (PCA). These include:

- Improper patient selection
- Inadequate monitoring
- Inadequate patient education
- Overriding of safety feature
- Medication mixup due to similarity in packaging
- Misprogramming of the pump
- Pump design flaw
- Inadequate staff training
- Prescribing errors

Case 4.15 illustrates a drug device error.

Case 4.15

An elderly patient awaiting surgery was prescribed morphine 2 mg/hr subcutaneously. The hospital's pain management protocol includes the use of a CADD Legacy pump with a 100-mL cassette containing 10 mg/mL of morphine. In programming the pump, the nurse entered 2 mL/hr instead of 2 mg/hr. This delivered a dose of 20 mg/hr. The error went unnoticed until the cassette was empty and the need for a cassette refill was questioned.

Note: This case is reprinted with permission from ISPM Canada. High alert drugs and infusion pumps: extra precautions required. ISMP Can Saf Bull. 2004;4(4):2.

Preventive Strategies for Drug Device Errors[10–12]

- Provide orientation and training for all users. All staff must be familiar with the various pumps, their settings, and their programming.
- Use standardized concentrations in order to minimize maneuvering tubing changes and possible confusion with various strengths of medications.
- Implement a policy requiring independent double checks.
- Use pumps and administration sets equipped with free-flow protection.
- Users should consider purchasing pumps with safety features such as software that provides safeguards against dosing and infusion-rate errors.
- Choose a pump with a lockout feature to prevent tampering by either the patient or the patient's visitors, especially in the case of pumps used at home.
- Caregivers should evaluate patients on PCA pumps and determine whether they need to manage their own pain and are capable of doing so. Patients should be properly educated on the pump's use.
- Ensure that caregivers recognize the signs and symptoms of opiate toxicity and withdrawal, the need to assess patients with minimal verbal or tactile stimulation, and have the ability to distinguish between oversedation and other pulmonary, neurological, or cardiovascular complications.
- Establish patient selection criteria for PCA. Candidates should have an appropriate level of consciousness and cognitive ability to manage their own pain.

LACK OF PATIENT EDUCATION/UNDERSTANDING

Patients can play a key role in preventing medication incidents. Patients who are well informed about their medications can serve as a last line of defense in preventing medication incidents. Many potential incidents can be identified during patient counseling. In fact, an educated patient can be the difference between an incident and a near miss. However, patients must feel empowered to ask questions about their therapy. They must also understand their responsibility to monitor their own therapy as much as possible. When patients take this control over their own health care, they can help avoid medication incidents.

However, many patients have difficulty understanding and acting upon the health information they are given. This is not a problem restricted only to uneducated, disabled, or elderly patients. According to the American Medical Association, more than 40% of patients with chronic illnesses are functionally illiterate. In addition, almost 25% of all adult Americans read at or below a grade 5 level, while medical information leaflets typically are written at a grade 10 level or higher.[13] According to the 2001 Census of the Population, Canadians reported more than 100 languages in completing the question on mother tongue.[14] Pharmacists should be aware of this trend and take steps to ensure that all patients receive and understand the information necessary to ensure appropriate use of their medication. This is especially important for patients who lack command of the official language. Even patients who speak

English fluently may still have difficulty interpreting written instructions that are vague.

Even when the pharmacist has provided the correct drug, with the correct directions to the correct patient, and provided all the appropriate information regarding its use, errors can still occur. Steps must, therefore, be taken to ensure that the patient fully understands the information provided regarding the use of the product. This is especially critical in dispensing drugs with a high potential for causing harm. For example, the ISMP has received reports of harm caused by the patient's inappropriate use of fentanyl transdermal patches.[15]

It is important for pharmacists to be aware of the safety issues surrounding the use of the fentanyl transdermal system and to ensure that patients and their caregivers are educated regarding its appropriate use.

Pharmacists must be aware of the following information[16,17] regarding the Duragesic patch:

- Serum fentanyl concentrations could theoretically increase by approximately one third for patients with a body temperature of 40°C owing to temperature-dependent increases in fentanyl release from the Duragesic system and increased skin permeability. Similarly, exposure of the application site to an external heat source such as a heating pad can increase drug absorption.
- Fentanyl is rapidly and extensively metabolized mainly by the cytochrome P450 3A4 isoenzyme system (CYP 3A4). Therefore, the concomitant use of fentanyl with potent CYP 3A4 inhibitors such as ritonavir, ketoconazole, and clarithromycin may result in an increase in fentanyl plasma concentrations, which could increase or prolong adverse drug effects and may cause potentially fatal respiratory depression.
- The use of damaged or cut patches can result in a rapid release of the contents of the patch and absorption of a potentially fatal dose of fentanyl.
- Fentanyl patches are intended for transdermal use on intact skin only; use on compromised skin can lead to increased exposure to fentanyl.
- Owing to the formation of a subcutaneous depot of fentanyl, the duration of the respiratory depressant effect of Duragesic may extend beyond the removal of the system.
- After removal of the Duragesic patch, serum fentanyl concentrations decline gradually, falling about 50% in approximately 17 hours.
- The following Web sites can be accessed for further information:
  www.janssen-ortho.com
  www.hc-sc.gc.ca/dhp-mps/medeff/index_e.html
  www.fda.gov/cder/drug/infopage/fentanyl/default.htm

The following information[16,17] should also be provided to patients and their caregivers to ensure safe use of the product.

- Duragesic patches should be applied to intact, nonirritated skin. Therefore, if the site of application must be cleansed prior to application of the patch, do not use soaps, alcohol, or any other agent that might irritate the skin or alter its characteristics. Cleanse the skin with clear water and allow the skin to dry completely prior to patch application.

- Duragesic patches should be applied immediately upon removal from the sealed package. The system should not be cut, divided, or damage in any way prior to its application since this leads to uncontrolled release of fentanyl.
- A new Duragesic patch should be applied on a different site *after* removal of the previous patch.
- The dose of fentanyl should never be adjusted unless recommended by the prescriber.
- If the patient develops a high fever while wearing the patch, he or she should contact the prescribing physician or the pharmacist for advice.
- Avoid exposing the patch application site to direct external heat sources, such as heating pads, electric blankets, heated water beds, heat lamps, hot water bottles, saunas, and hot whirlpool spa baths.
- Be aware of the signs and symptoms of fentanyl overdose and seek medical attention immediately should these signs and symptoms be noted. They include trouble breathing or shallow breathing; tiredness, extreme sleepiness or sedation; inability to think, talk, or walk normally; and feeling faint, dizzy, or confused.
- Keep the patches in a secure place out of the reach of children owing to the high risk of fatal respiratory depression should such a patch be used by a child.
- Used systems should be folded so that the adhesive side of the system adheres to itself and then flushed down the toilet immediately upon removal. Unused systems that are no longer needed should be returned to the pharmacy for safe disposal as soon as possible. Otherwise, they may be discarded by removing the left-over patches from their protective pouches and removing the protective liners. Then the patches may be folded in half and flushed down the toilet. Do not flush the pouch or protective liner.
- The patient should inform all health care practitioners providing medical or dental care that he or she is currently using a fentanyl patch.

Case 4.16 is another example where the patient's lack of understanding led to a drug administration error.

Case 4.16

An arthritic patient was given a written prescription for methotrexate with the instructions "Take as directed." The prescription was taken to the local pharmacy for filling and dispensed correctly. The patient received the methotrexate tablets and began to take three 2.5-mg tablets (7.5 mg) daily.

Approximately 2 weeks later, the patient was admitted to the hospital for an unrelated diagnosis. Upon being questioned regarding his medication use, the patient indicated that he was currently taking 7.5 mg of methotrexate each day. An order was, therefore, written for the patient to continue taking 7.5 mg methotrexate daily while he was in the hospital.

Two days later, in reviewing the patient's medication regimen, a hospital pharmacist identified the patient's daily dosage of methotrexate as potentially erroneous. The pharmacist spoke with the patient, who assured her that the dose was

7.5 mg each day. Still not satisfied, the pharmacist contacted the community pharmacy where the prescription had been filled. The dispensing pharmacist indicated that the directions for use was written "Take as directed." The hospital pharmacist then contacted the prescriber, who confirmed that the dosage should be 7.5 mg once weekly.

The patient's dosage was, therefore, adjusted. Fortunately the patient suffered no known ill effects.

The hospital pharmacist deserved to be commended for her diligence, which prevented serious harm.

Possible Contributory Factors

- The prescription was written with the instructions "Take as directed."
- The patient forgot the verbal instructions given by the physician.
- The dispensing pharmacist did not confirm the patient's understanding of how the medication should be taken.
- The patient was admitted to the hospital during a weekend. This created barriers to obtaining a complete medication history as well as contacting the patient's community pharmacy and prescribing physician.

Preventive Strategies for Lack of Patient Education

- Whenever possible, educate prescibers about the potential problems associated with vague instructions such as "Take as directed."
- Confirm the patient's understanding of the dosage regimen. Ask the patient, "How were you told to take this medication?" If the patient is unsure or indicates an unusual dosage, contact the prescriber for clarification.
- Provide the patient with clearly written instructions on when and how to take the medication. For once-weekly dosing, indicate a specific day of the week. The directions for use may, therefore, be written as "Take 3 tablets every Thursday."
- On admission to hospital, the patient's community pharmacy should be contacted for a complete medication history.
- Make every effort to clarify any information that does not seem right.
- Upon discharge, the patient's pharmacy should also be contacted to update the patient's medication regimen. If this is not possible, the patient should be given a complete written record to be taken to his pharmacy.

FAILED COMMUNICATION WITH PATIENTS

Patients must be willing to ask a question when something does not seem right. Unfortunately, patients are at times hesitant to speak up despite receiving an unexpected change in drug therapy. Most patients have a high level of trust in their doctors and pharmacists and may, therefore, see it as inappropriate to question whether they were given the correct drug. Patients may also see their doctors and pharmacists as authoritative individuals and may, therefore, feel reluctant to questioning them.

As a result, patients may consider other explanations for the change in therapy. They may assume that the physician simply forgot to inform them of the change or that the pharmacist provided a different brand of their medication. Cases 4.17 and 4.18 show how necessary it is to have effective communication with patients.

Case 4.17

Mrs. O arrived at her local community pharmacy for a refill of her hydrochlorothiazide 25-mg tablets, which were previously ordered and ready to be picked up. The pharmacist, who has known Mrs. O for over 30 years, chatted with her for approximately 5 minutes. While chatting, he reached into the "O to R" bin and retrieved what was thought to be Mrs. O's prescription and gave it to her.

Later that day, Mr. P arrived at the pharmacy to pick up a refill of his oxybutynin 5-mg tablets. A search of the pharmacy failed to locate the prescription. As a result of a printer problem earlier that day, it was assumed that the prescription label did not print. A second label was, therefore, printed and the oxybutynin was prepared and given to Mr. P.

A few days later, while checking the prescription bins to identify prescriptions that were not picked up, a technician located Mrs. O's prescription. However, the pharmacist recalled chatting with Mrs. O and giving her the medication. It was, therefore, assumed that as a result of the printer problems, the prescription must have been prepared twice.

Approximately 3 months later, Mrs. O returned to the pharmacy with Mr P's prescription vial for a refill of her medication. On attempting to process the prescription refill, the technician noticed that Mr. P's prescription was filled the previous day. The pharmacist was, therefore, summoned to take Mrs. O to the private counseling area.

Upon questioning Mrs. O, it was discovered that she had been taking oxybutynin 5-mg tablets each day for the preceding 3 months. She did not question the pharmacist despite the different color and appearance of the tablets.

The doctor was contacted and informed of the error. The patient was then sent to the physician for an assessment. Fortunately no ill effects were observed.

Possible Contributory Factors

- The pharmacist was distracted and did not check the name on the prescription bag before giving it to Mrs. O.
- The cashier did not look at the patient's name when ringing up the prescription.
- The patient did not read the prescription label.
- The patient assumed that the pharmacist had given her a different brand of hydrochlorothiazide.

Case 4.18

John Westheimer, a 67-year-old patient, presented a prescription for 60 hydro-chlorothiazide 25-mg tablets at his local community pharmacy for filling. Shortly thereafter, a second patient, Les Reimer, requested a refill of his Lipitor tablets. Both prescriptions were filled accurately.

Approximately 10 minutes later, the technician called out for Les Reimer. Mr. Westheimer, who had a poor command of spoken English, assumed that his name was being mispronounced and came forward. The technician, therefore, proceeded to ring up the prescription. Mr. Westheimer seemed surprised at the price of the prescription, but being apprehensive about his communication skills, chose to pay what asked. Counseling did not take place since it was assumed that the patient had taken Lipitor before.

Later that day, Mr. Reimer returned to pick up his prescription. It was at this time that the error was detected. When he was contacted, Mr. Westheimer had already taken one dose of the incorrect drug. Fortunately there were no identified ill effects.

Preventive Strategies for Failed Communication

- In giving out prescriptions, check the patient's name and a second piece of information, such as the patient's address or phone number, to verify that the correct medication is being given out.
- Make patient counseling a component of the dispensing of all new prescriptions and refills as appropriate.
- Patient counseling provides the opportunity to verify the accuracy of dispensing, and it provides confirmation that the patient understands the proper use of the medication. At a minimum, patients should know:
  - The name of the medication (both brand and generic names)
  - The purpose of each medication
  - How to take the medication
  - When to take it
  - How it works
  - What it looks like
  - How to store it
  - What to do if doses are missed
  - Potential side effects and how to handle them
- Review the patient's medication history to identify changes in therapy, dosage, and frequency. Discuss and confirm these changes with the patient.
- Ask the patient to repeat the information provided to confirm his or her understanding to you.
- During patient counseling, consider opening the prescription vial, thereby enabling both you and the patient to take a final look at the medication.
- Encourage patients to ask questions, especially whenever something seems wrong or unusual with the medication.

- Assess the patient's level of understanding of the information that is provided through effective dialogue. Confirm what the patient already knows through open-ended questions and identify gaps in knowledge and opportunities for reinforcement.
- Follow-up with the patient to ensure that he or she is taking the medication as prescribed and that there are no drug-related problems.
- Suggest that patients keep written records of their current prescription medications and over-the-counter products.
- When language barriers are identified, consider translating written information as your computer software permits.
- Make use of signs and symbols as appropriate.
- Use other staff members as interpreters if they speak the same language as the patient.
- Watch for and react to verbal and nonverbal cues from the patient that may indicate something is wrong.

SUMMARY

Some of the most common causes of medication error are discussed in this chapter. These include failed written and verbal communication, look-alike/sound-alike drug names, calculation errors, and lack of patient education.

In the following chapters, underlying root causes and prevention strategies to medication error are discussed.

Reflective Questions

1. Use examples of medication incidents that have occurred in your practice and identify three or more contributory factors for each incident.
2. For each incident identified in question 1, describe prevention strategies that could be implemented to prevent the incident from recurring.
3. Identify one look-alike/sound-alike drug that has contributed to a medication incident. Discuss prevention strategies to prevent this incident in the future.
4. Develop a strategy to discourage the use of abbreviations and symbols in your practice.

REFERENCES

1. Medication errors blamed on handwriting, tired nurses, CBC Winnipeg. Available at: http://winnipeg.cbc.ca/regional/servlet/View?filename=mb_mederrors20030415. Accessed May 24, 2004.
2. Einerson A, Bailey B, Koren G. Pregnancy outcome of women exposed to pinaverium due to a dispensing error. *Ann Pharmacother.* 1999;33:112–113.
3. Reminyl renamed Razadyne in U.S. to support patient safety. Available at www.razadyne.com/html/raz/pd_main.xml?article=media_releases_20050411.jspf. Accessed May 17, 2005.

4. ISPM. Lessons lost by the global pharmaceutical industry. *ISMP Med Saf Alert.* 2001;6(8):1.
5. Caverly WM. Improving efficiencies and reducing medication. Part 2: Product placement. The Efficient Pharmacy 2000;3(3):4.
6. Dorland's Illustrated Medical Dictionary. Philadelphia: Saunders; 1994:1520.
7. Lesar TS, Briceland L, Stein DS. Factors related to errors in medication prescribing. *JAMA.* 1997:277:312–317.
8. Abraham C. Dosage errors imperil children: study. *Globe Mail,* April 11, 2002.
9. Rolfe S, Harper NJ. Ability of hospital doctors to calculate drug doses. *BMJ.* 1995; 310:1173–1174.
10. Health risks associated with use of infusion pumps—notice to hospitals. April 16, 2004. Available at: www.hc-sc.gc.ca/hpfb-dgpsa/tpd-dpt/infusion_pumps_nth_e.html. Accessed September 2, 2007.
11. How to prevent errors, part 2. Safety issues with patient controlled analgesia. *ISMP Med Saf Alert.* 2003;8(15).
12. ISPM. High alert drugs and infusion pumps: extra precautions required. *ISMP Can Saf Bull.* 2004;4(4):2.
13. American Medical Association. Ad Hoc Committee on Health Literacy for the Council on Scientific Affairs. Health literacy: report of the Council on Scientific Affairs. *JAMA.* 1999;281:552–557.
14. 2001 Census: analysis series, Profile of languages in Canada: English, French and many others. Statistics Canada 2002.
15. New fentanyl warnings: more needed to protect patients. *ISMP Med Saf Alert.* 2005; 10(16):1–3.
16. Duragesic Product Monograph. Version date September 8, 2005.
17. FDA Public Health Advisory. Safety warnings regarding use of fentanyl transdermal (skin) patches. Available at: www.fda.gov/cder/drug/advisory/fentanyl.htm. Accessed January 31, 2007.

Chapter 5

Underlying Root Causes and Preventive Strategies

Objectives

After completing this chapter, the reader will be able to:

- Understand the underlying root causes of medication incidents in pharmacy practice
- Identify similar situations in pharmacy practice that could lead to medication incidents
- Identify preventive strategies for underlying root causes of medication incidents
- Understand human factors and environmental factors implicated in medication incidents
- Apply the knowledge gained to your current practice with a view to prevent future incidents
- Identify Web sites that can be key resources for error prevention strategies

In addition to the immediate causes of medication incidents discussed in the previous chapter, we have seen that tracing occurrences back to the root cause may identify several system breakdowns acting as contributory factors. A systems analysis approach to medication incidents helps to determine a number of contributory factors that go deeper than just what occurred during the drug dispensing process. In this chapter we discuss psychological and human factors, dispensing process, manufacturer issues, seamless care, pharmacy workload, environment, and organizational issues.

PSYCHOLOGICAL AND HUMAN FACTORS

Psychologists have studied human cognition in an effort to understand why we make errors and how to prevent them. Grasha and O'Neill[1] suggest that prescription errors are related to cognitive system failures. These may include failures in sensory memory, deficiencies in the storage and retrieval of information in short- and long-term memory, working memory overload, attention deficits, inadequate retrieval and monitoring of sensorimotor scripts, and possessing insufficient knowledge.

A better understanding of the human cognitive system is key to the prevention of medication incidents.

Automatic and Problem-Solving Mode

There are two modes of mental functioning: automatic and problem-solving.[2] The automatic mode is unconscious and effortless and the state of most of our mental functioning for things such as eating or driving. This mode serves us well until there is a change that we need to notice. An example would be setting out in your car to go grocery shopping but finding yourself driving to work instead. The problem-solving mode takes the form of intense mental activity involving the application of rules and use of stored knowledge. It is conscious, slow, and sequential and therefore more difficult.[2]

Slips are incidents that occur when our minds are on automatic mode. They stem basically from a failure of attention or perception. Usually they occur because we are distracted or not paying full attention or our thought process is lost. For example, a pharmacist may check a number of prescriptions and have no memory of doing so because he or she was in automatic mode.

Diversion of attention can also be caused by environmental factors such as noise, heat, or motion and physiological factors such as fatigue, sleep loss, alcohol, drugs, illness, and hunger. Psychological factors such as boredom, frustration, anxiety, and anger can be triggered by internal or external factors such as overwork, interpersonal relations, and other forms of stress.[2]

Errors that occur when the pharmacist is in problem-solving mode are knowledge-based mistakes. Error occurs when we are faced with situations where we have no programmed solution because we lack the needed knowledge or have misinterpreted the problem.

Studies of medication incidents have found that when pharmacists' actions were a major contributory factor in an incident, they generally were due to a lack of current knowledge (e.g., a drug interaction with a new medication, a recently uncovered drug interaction, or a new drug that is not recognized and therefore is confused with a known drug of a similar name). Lack of knowledge can also apply to the prescriber, who may also confuse names and dosages or be unaware of drug interactions and contraindications.

It has been noted by the Institute for Safe Medication Practices that use of outdated and incorrect references—including reference texts, journal articles, and charts—is a contributory factor to medication errors.[3]

Confirmation Bias

Many medication errors can be attributed to human factors such as cognitive functioning. The principle of confirmation bias has been identified as a possible contributory factor in a number of errors.

Confirmation bias describes the tendency to look for and interpret information in a way that confirms one's preconceptions and to ignore or not look for contradictory information. We therefore tend to "see" what is in our memory or what we believe to be true. When a pharmacist cannot read a poorly written prescription, he or she will call the prescriber for clarification. However, if the pharmacist believes that the prescription is being read correctly, he or she will tend to accept what the prescription appears to say.

Confirmation bias leads us to see information that confirms our expectation and ignore information that contradicts it. Recent graduates read written prescriptions and labels carefully because they are not yet familiar with drug names and packages. However, a more experienced pharmacist is more likely to read the first few letters of a drug name and fill in the gaps based on previous knowledge and memory. Figure 5.1 illustrates this point.

Aoccdrnig to rscheearch at Cmabrigde Uinervtisy, it deosn't mttaer in waht oredr the ltteers in a wrod are, the olny iprmoetnt tihng is taht the frist and lsat ltteer be at the rghit pclae. The rset can be a total mses and you can sitll raed it wouthit porbelm.

FIGURE 5.1 Filling in the gaps.

If two look-alike drugs have the same strength, the pharmacy technician may see the wrong one. This is why knowledge is so important—if the pharmacist or technician does not know that another possible name exists, he or she will not even consider looking for it.

Examples of confirmation bias are illustrated in Case 5.1 and Case 5.2, which occurred in Canada.

Case 5.1

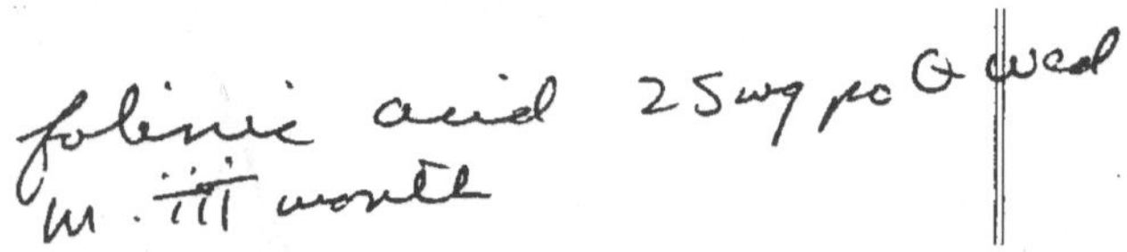

The prescription shown here was presented to a pharmacy technician for processing. The prescription was entered into the computer as folic acid 5 mg, with the directions to take five tablets every Wednesday. The physician had used a synonym, folinic acid, for the intended prescription of calcium folinate. Unlike folic acid, calcium folinate is administered to patients to diminish the toxicity of methotrexate. It can also be used for pretreatment followed by 5-fluorouracil to prolong survival in the palliative treatment of patients with advanced colorectal cancer.[4] Upon checking the prescription, the pharmacist did not detect the error.

The pharmacist began to provide patient counseling but was interrupted by the patient, who said, "The prescription is not for folic acid. This is the second time that this error has been made."

Possible Contributory Factors

- The terms "folic acid" and "folinic acid" look alike.
- Both folic acid and calcium folinate are available in the same strength (5 mg) and dosage form (tablet).
- Many pharmacists and technicians are unaware of the use of "folinic acid" as a synonym for "calcium folinate."
- Pharmacists and technicians are familiar with the drug folic acid. As a result, in reading a prescription for folinic acid, they are more likely to see what is most familiar to them.

Case 5.2

The prescription shown here was presented to a pharmacy technician for processing. The technician interpreted and entered the prescription into the computer as Tanacet. The patient was informed that the product was not in stock and would be ordered from the supplier for pickup the following day.

The patient returned the next day for the medication. The technician then retrieved Tanacet from the order, labeled the product, and gave it to the pharmacist for checking. Upon checking the prescription, the pharmacist found that the prescription was actually written for Tramacet and not Tanacet.

Possible Contributory Factors

- Tramacet and Tanacet can sound alike and look alike.
- The technician was familiar with the product Tanacet and was not familiar with the new product Tramacet. The technician therefore "saw" what was known.
- The same technician completed all of the technical functions in processing the prescription, including accepting the written prescription, entering it into the computer, ordering the product, and labeling it. A second pair of eyes might have identified the error at an earlier stage in the process.

Preventive Strategies for Confirmation Bias

- Educate all pharmacy staff about the potential for a mixup between folic acid and folinic acid.
- Advise prescribers of the potential for error when the term "folinic acid" is used to prescribe calcium folinate. Discourage the use of the term "folinic acid."
- Always double-check prescribed dosages for appropriateness.
- Whenever a medication error or potential error is identified, ensure that all pharmacy staff is informed. Develop strategies to make sure that the same error does not recur in your pharmacy. This may include the addition of notes to the patient profile and both drug files that can serve as alert flags.
- Have "two sets of eyes" review each prescription. In asking for a second opinion, do not offer your review until you have heard the other opinion. For example, show the prescription to the second person and ask, "What do you see here?"
- Maintain a list of problematic drug pairs and educate all pharmacy staff about the potential for error.
- Place auxiliary labels in front of these products to alert staff.

DISPENSING PROCESS

During the dispensing process, there are many stages when things can go wrong and thus contribute to a medication incident. A number of critical steps have been identified in the dispensing process that require focused attention.[3]

1. Review and assessment of prescription
2. Computer data entry
3. Review of patient profile
4. Assessment of computer alerts
5. Verification of questions with the prescriber
6. Selection of medication (in computer and from shelf)
7. Verification of expiry date
8. Counting or measuring medication
9. Affixing label
10. Double-checking prescription
11. Returning stock to proper location
12. Patient counseling and taking of history

Examples of errors that can occur during the dispensing process include computer entry errors, allergy-related issues, tablet/vial mixups, returning medications to the stock bottle, transferring prescriptions, and drug stability/storage. Cases 5.3 to 5.13 describe a variety of incidents that can occur in the dispensing process.

Computer Entry: Drug Selection

Case 5.3

An elderly patient took the following prescription to her local pharmacy for processing.

Prednisone 5 mg
Sig: Take 2 tablets twice daily
Dispense: 28

In entering the drug name into the computer, the pharmacy technician, in error, selected prednisone 50 mg. A second technician counted the tablets and labeled the vial but did not detect the data entry error. The pharmacist also checked and signed the prescription without detecting the error. Prednisone 50-mg tablets were therefore dispensed to the patient with label instructions to take 2 tablets twice daily (i.e., 200 mg daily) instead of the prescribed 20 mg daily, a 10-fold overdose.

The patient took the medication home and attempted to take the first dose. Fortunately, she had previously taken prednisone 5-mg tablets and therefore detected the change in the tablets' appearance. She then read the prescription label, identified the error, and contacted the pharmacy.

Possible Contributory Factors

- While entering prescriptions into the computer, the pharmacy technician was constantly interrupted by patients approaching the pharmacy counter.
- The pharmacy technician initially entered an abbreviated form of the drug name into the computer and then highlighted and selected the incorrect strength of prednisone from the list of available strengths.
- The second pharmacy technician assumed that the printed prescription label was correct and therefore prepared prednisone 50 mg.
- A minimal amount of patient counseling took place because the patient had previously taken prednisone.

Case 5.4

A mother presented a prescription for Cortisporin Ophthalmic Drops for her 8-year-old son at her local pharmacy. The technician correctly entered the prescription into the computer. However, a second technician inadvertently selected Cortisporin Otic Drops from the shelf. The prescription label was placed over most of the box, making it difficult for the pharmacist to detect the error. The otic solution was therefore dispensed.

After the first drop was instilled into the patient's eye, he "screamed" in discomfort. The error was detected after the mother called the pharmacy to discuss the child's reaction.

Possible Contributory Factors

- Similarity in Cortisporin products.
- The packages of the two products are similar in size and shape.
- The products are stored next to each other.
- Neither the technician nor the pharmacist compared the Drug Identification Number (Canada). The National Drug Code (NDC) system is used in the United States.
- The prescription label covered most of the information on the Cortisporin box.

Computer Entry: Expired Prescriptions

Patients with chronic medical conditions often experience a change in drug therapy over time. Failure to deactivate the "old" prescription can result in a number of "active" prescriptions with the potential for error. In addition, patients often present new prescriptions for medications for which there are valid refill authorizations remaining on file. This results in the existence of multiple "valid" prescriptions simultaneously. The following two cases, 5.5 and 5.6, illustrate these circumstances.

Case 5.5

A 70-year-old patient had been taking Norvasc 5-mg tablets once daily for an extended period of time. Following a checkup visit with her physician, her dosage was increased to 10 mg once daily and a written prescription was given to the patient to reflect the increase in dose.

The patient took her prescription to her community pharmacy for filling. However, she informed the pharmacist that she had recently filled a prescription for the 5-mg tablets and questioned whether it would be appropriate to continue taking the 5-mg tablets that she had at home until they were finished. The pharmacist approved, telling her to "double up" the tablets. The new prescription was therefore logged for dispensing at a future date.

However, in error, the patient continued to take one 5-mg tablet each day. In addition, once having used up the the tablets, the patient contacted the pharmacy and asked for a refill. The pharmacy technician then selected the last prescription for Norvasc that had been dispensed (i.e., the 5-mg tablets). Since one previously authorized refill remained on file, an additional 3-month supply of Norvasc 5-mg tablets was dispensed, and she continued to take a tablet a day. Approximately 3 months later, the patient asked for another refill of her Norvasc tablets. The pharmacy technician again selected the 5-mg strength, and since no authorized refills remained on file, the physician was contacted for the authority to dispense. A check of the patient's medical records indicated that the dose of Norvasc had been increased approximately 5 months earlier. The physician therefore contacted the pharmacy and asked that the 10-mg tablets be dispensed.

Possible Contributory Factors

- A breakdown in communication between pharmacist and patient.
- On receiving the new prescription for Norvasc 10 mg tablets, the pharmacy had no system for deactivating previous prescriptions that should no longer be dispensed.
- A lack of system in place to identify the presence of logged prescriptions on file when prescriptions are being refilled.

Case 5.6

A 45-year-old patient approached a pharmacy technician at his local community pharmacy and requested a refill of his Paxil 20-mg tablets. The technician checked his medication history to identify the prescription. Observing that there were no refills remaining on his last prescription, the technician scanned the remainder of the patient's profile to see if there were any refills remaining on previously filled prescriptions for Paxil 20 mg. She noticed that another prescription was on file with two refill authorizations unused. This prescription was therefore selected for filling. The prescription was filled accurately for Paxil 20 mg and dispensed.

However, since the time the previous prescription had been filled, the patient had changed doctors; the new doctor increased his daily dosage from 20 mg (one tablet daily) to 40 mg (two tablets daily). Without reading the prescription label, the patient continued to take his current dosage of two tablets in the morning. After finishing his medication prematurely, the patient read the label and identified that the wrong prescription had been filled. On returning to the pharmacy, the patient was very upset and shouted that he was given "the wrong prescription, with the wrong dosage, the wrong quantity, and the wrong doctor."

Possible Contributory Factors

- The patient did not provide a specific prescription number in requesting the refill.
- The technician did not take steps to ensure that the prescription selected was identical to the last prescription filled.
- The pharmacy had no system in place to inactivate "old" prescriptions that are no longer valid.
- There were no guidelines in place at the pharmacy regarding the filling of "old" prescriptions with "valid" refills.
- In checking the prescription, there was no information available to the pharmacist to indicate the change in dosage, doctor, and quantity as compared with the last prescription processed for Paxil.

Computer Entry: Sig Codes

Pharmacists may be less vigilant when checking the refill of a prescription because it is often assumed that the information previously entered was correct. However in some instances, the information may have been changed since the original prescription was filled as illustrated in Case 5.7.

Case 5.7

A 50-year-old patient took the following prescription to her pharmacy for filling.

Baclofen 10 mg
Sig: Take half a tablet up to three times daily.
May increase the dose to a maximum of one tablet
three times daily if needed.
Dispense: 30

On entering the prescription into the computer, the pharmacy technician encountered some difficulty entering the directions for use owing to the limited space available. However, the software did permit the creation of expanded sig files with the use of unique codes.

The technician selected the patient's name as a unique code in creating the expanded directions-for-use file. The Baclofen tablets were therefore prepared and labeled correctly.

One week later, the patient returned to the pharmacy with the following prescription.

Tegretol Chewable 100 mg
Sig: Chew one tablet twice daily. Increase each dose by one tablet until
pain is relieved or to a maximum of 12 tablets per day.
Dispense: 100

On this occasion, another technician entered the patient's code to create an expanded sig file. Upon entering the code, the directions for use of Baclofen appeared on the screen. Unaware of the implications, the technician overrode the directions for use to those for the Tegretol Chewable tablets. The Tegretol Chewable tablets were therefore prepared and labeled correctly.

Approximately a month later, the patient asked for a refill of her Baclofen tablets. However, because of the change made to the sig file, the Baclofen label read "Chew one tablet twice daily. Increase each dose by one tablet until pain is relieved or to a maximum of twelve tablets per day." Upon checking the prescription, the pharmacist did not detect the labeling error. Fortunately the patient was aware of the correct directions for taking Baclofen.

Possible Contributory Factors

- Limited space available to enter an expanded sig.
- Incomplete training of dispensary staff.
- The computer software permits the operator to change information contained in files, which can affect a number of other prescriptions, thereby jeopardizing patient safety.

Preventive Strategies for Computer Entry Errors

- In retrieving products for dispensing, always read the original prescription first, select the product, and then compare the product selected with that on the computer-generated hard copy. This is a key step in identifying input errors.
- Minimize interruptions when you are performing key functions such as computer entry and the checking of prescriptions.
- Computer entry should be delegated to a well-trained pharmacy technician.
- In checking prescriptions, always consider the appropriateness of the drug, dose, and dosage form.
- Check all components of a refill prescription, including directions for use.
- Ensure that all dispensary staff are appropriately trained. Review the implications of overriding the translation of codes. For example, if the letter "T" is a code for teaspoon, there would be serious implications if it were changed to tablespoon. This is especially important for newly hired or temporary staff, as the translation of a specific code may vary depending on the computer system.
- Discuss with your software vendor the need to restrict changes to files that can affect other prescriptions and hence other patients.
- Contact your software vendor to discuss the addition of system alerts to identify the presence of a related logged prescription when a refill prescription is being processed.
- Provide clear verbal and written communication to patients, especially when there is a change in dosage or therapy.
- Use a highlighter to indicate changes.
- Ask the patient to repeat the information provided to confirm his or her understanding.
- Whenever there is a change in dosage or drug therapy, establish a system to deactivate all previously dispensed medications that should no longer be dispensed. Add a notation to link these deactivated prescriptions to the new prescription.
- Educate pharmacy team members of the dangers of using "old" prescriptions.
- If an "old" prescription must be used, ensure that the dosage, etc., is identical to the current regimen.
- When you receive a new prescription for a drug that has valid refills remaining on another prescription, consider contacting the prescriber to clarify the

status of the refills. It is usually not the prescriber's intent to have a number of valid prescriptions running simultaneously.

- In scanning the list of products in the computer, be careful to select the correct product and package size.
- Always check the patient's history. This can be a great tool in identifying changes in drug therapy or potential medication errors.
- When you are counseling a patient, first ask "What did the doctor tell you about this medication?"
- When they are labeling products, pharmacy technicians should avoid covering critical information before the prescription is checked by the pharmacist.

Allergy-Related Issues

Case 5.8

A 40-year-old patient with a known allergy to cephalosporin received a prescription for Ceftin 500 mg to be taken three times daily. The patient took the prescription to his regular pharmacy for filling.

Upon entering the prescription into the computer, the technician received a clinical warning regarding the potential for an allergic reaction. The technician attempted to ask the pharmacist for advice. However, the pharmacist was on the telephone speaking to a physician regarding another patient. Not knowing the significance of the alert and in an effort to prevent a delay in the processing of prescriptions, the technician decided to override the alert by simply striking a key. The technician intended to speak with the pharmacist at the end of the phone call but forgot. The pharmacist checked the prescription but did not notice the warning regarding the patient's allergy. The Ceftin was dispensed and the pharmacist provided counseling on the use of the medication.

On arriving at home, the patient decided to read the written information that was provided and became alarmed after reading that "this medication is a cephalosporin." The patient therefore contacted the pharmacy and was very upset that he was given a drug to which he was allergic.

Preventive Strategies for Allergy Related Issues

- When you are entering patient information into the computer, ensure the patient's allergies or "no known allergies" has been entered.
- Develop a system of differentiating between true allergies and intolerance to medication.
- Ensure that the information is accurately coded.
- When you are receiving verbal prescriptions, ask the prescriber about the patient's allergies.
- Take all allergy computer warnings seriously. Never assume that an allergy warning is insignificant.
- Consider restricting the overriding of allergy alerts to pharmacists only.

- Pharmacy technicians should request a pharmacist's intervention before an allergy prompt is overridden.
- Screen all allergy prompts by asking the patient the nature of his or her allergy and then document this information.
- Consider cross-sensitivity reactions that may occur with specific drugs.
- Document any discussion you have with the prescriber or patient.
- During the counseling session, verify that the allergy information is current and that there have been no changes since the patient's last visit.
- Contact your software vendor to ask that allergy warnings be prominently printed on the computer-generated hard copy.

Tablet/Vial Mixups

Case 5.9

Following a routine checkup visit with their physician, 83-year-old Mr. Smith and 80-year-old Mrs. Smith were given the following prescriptions:
Mr. Smith:

Metformin 500 mg

Sig: 1 b.i.d.

Dispense: 100

Mrs. Smith:

Tenormin 50 mg

Sig: 1 o.d.

Dispense: 60

No substitution

The prescriptions were taken to the Smiths' regular pharmacy for filling. Mrs. Smith asked that brand-name Tenormin be dispensed. Both drugs were prepared and labeled correctly by the pharmacy technician. However, on checking the prescription, the pharmacist detected an error in the third-party billing, which resulted in Mrs. Smith being asked to pay a higher than usual copayment. The technician was therefore asked to rebill the third-party insurance by entering the appropriate intervention code, which would indicate that the physician had requested that brand-Tenormin be dispensed. The third-party insurance therefore paid for the Tenormin.

A new receipt and label were generated for the Tenormin prescription. However, in error, the label was placed on the vial containing Mr. Smith's metformin tablets. On rechecking the prescription, the pharmacist did not detect the labeling error. As a result, the pharmacist dispensed Mrs. Smith's Tenormin appropriately labeled and Mr. Smith's metformin labeled as Mrs. Smith's Tenormin.

A few days later, Mrs. Smith opened the vial labeled Tenormin and identified the content as her husband's metformin. She then called the pharmacy to report that she had been given her husband's tablets in error.

Possible Contributory Factors

- Mr. and Mrs. Smith's prescriptions were both prepared by the same technician at the same time.
- Mrs. Smith has coverage with two third-party insurance plans. As a result, the technician found the procedure for billing brand-name Tenormin to be complex.
- The prescription had been checked previously; therefore, on rechecking the prescription, the pharmacist did not compare the contents of the vial with the information on the label.
- The delay in processing of the prescription likely placed undue stress on the pharmacist to complete the checking of the prescription quickly.

Preventive Strategies for Tablet/Vial Mixups

- In checking prescriptions, perform a visual check of the contents of the prescription vial. Carefully compare the contents of the vial with the information on the prescription label. This is especially critical if the prescription vial is left unlabeled for any period of time during the dispensing process.
- It is advisable to process each patient's prescription separately.
- When changes are made to a prescription, recheck all components to confirm accuracy.
- Ensure that all staff are appropriately trained on third-party billing procedures.
- During patient counseling, open the prescription vial, thereby enabling both you and the patient to take a final look at the medication. This is a critical step, as many dispensing errors can be detected at this point.

Returning Medications to the Stock Bottle

For a variety of reasons, prepared medications not dispensed to patients may be returned to stock. This critical step, if taken lightly, can be a factor in dispensing errors that may result in patient harm, as seen in Case 5.10.

Case 5.10

A 72-year-old patient received the following prescription upon discharge from the hospital:

Prednisone 30 mg AM for 4 days,
then decrease by 5 mg every 5th day
Lorazepam 1 mg
Sig: ud
Dispense: 30

The prescription was taken to the local community pharmacy for filling. Upon reading the prescription, the pharmacy technician determined that a total of 99 prednisone 5-mg tablets would be required for the course of therapy. That is, 6, 6, 6, 6, 5, 5, 5, 5, 5, 4, 4, 4, 4, 4, etc. The technician then used an electronic tablet counter to correctly count and label 99 prednisone 5-mg tablets. Thirty lorazepam 1-mg tablets were also counted and labeled separately.

On checking the prescription, the pharmacist determined that only 84 prednisone 5-mg tablets would be required to complete the course of therapy. That is, 6, 6, 6, 6, 5, 5, 5, 5, 4, 4, 4, 4, etc.

On being asked to recount the prednisone tablets, the technician decided to first return the 99 prednisone 5-mg tablets to the original stock bottle. However, in error, the technician poured the prednisone 5-mg tablets into the lorazepam 1-mg stock bottle. She then poured what was now a mixture of prednisone 5-mg tablets and lorazepam 1-mg tablets into the tablet counter until it recorded 84. This mixture of tablets was then placed in a prescription vial and labeled as 84 prednisone 5-mg tablets. The pharmacist did not detect the error; therefore the patient received the 30 lorazepam 1-mg tablets labeled correctly and the mixture of prednisone 5-mg tablets and lorazepam 1-mg tablets labeled as prednisone 5 mg. On arriving home, the patient opened the vial labeled prednisone 5 mg to take her first dose and identified the presence of two different tablets in the vial. By contacting the pharmacy immediately to report the error, the patient not only protected herself from potential harm but also prevented future patients from receiving a similar mixture of tablets. Although patient harm did not occur, the patient's confidence in the pharmacy's ability to provide appropriate care was diminished.

Possible Contributory Factors

- The stock bottles containing prednisone 5 mg and lorazepam 1 mg came from the same manufacturer and were identical in size, shape, and color.
- The prednisone tablets were returned to a stock bottle without first being appropriately checked.
- Despite the differences in shape and size between prednisone 5-mg and lorazepam 1-mg tablets, the technician did not detect the error when she was pouring the tablets into the prescription vial.

Preventive Strategies for Returning Medication to Stock

- Be extremely careful in returning tablets to original stock bottles. If tablets must be returned to a stock bottle, a minimum of two staff must independently check to confirm that the correct drug is being returned. Of course the tablets must have originated from the same lot number found on the stock bottle.
- In checking prescriptions, open the prescription vial to confirm the identity of the tablets being dispensed.
- During patient counseling, consider opening the prescription vial in the presence of the patient, thereby enabling both you and the patient to take a final look at the medication.

Transferring Prescriptions

Patients often ask that their pharmacist contact another pharmacy to "transfer" their prescriptions. Although the information provided by the transferring pharmacy is usually accurate, there is also the potential for the transfer of incorrect information, as the shown in Cases 5.11 and 5.12.

Case 5.11

A 55-year-old patient asked for a refill of her prescription for Miacalcin, which was originally filled at another pharmacy. The pharmacist called the other pharmacy for a "transfer" of the prescription. On receiving the transfer, the pharmacist was given the directions for use as "one spray into each nostril daily." Being familiar with the usual dosage for Miacalcin, the receiving pharmacist questioned the directions. The transferring pharmacist rechecked the computer and repeated the same directions. Still not satisfied, the pharmacist insisted that the original prescription be retrieved. After checking the original written prescription, the directions for use as written by the prescriber were confirmed to be "one spray intranasally daily." Although the patient had used twice the recommended dosage for approximately a month, no ill effects were observed.

Possible Contributory Factors

- Unlike Miacalcin, most nasal sprays are administered into each nostril.
- The pharmacist who initially dispensed the Miacalcin was unfamiliar with the dosage regimen of the product and therefore entered incorrect directions for use in the computer.

Case 5.12

An ophthalmologist prescribed Timoptic 0.5% ophthalmic drops with the instructions to instill one drop into each eye twice daily. The 70-year-old glaucoma patient took the written prescription to his regular pharmacy for filling. In error, the pharmacy technician entered Timoptic XE 0.5% with the same directions to instill twice daily. A second technician read the computer-generated hard copy and therefore retrieved Timoptic XE 0.5% from the shelf. The pharmacist also failed to detect the error in checking the prescription. The patient therefore received Timoptic XE 0.5% with the instructions to instill it twice daily, although the recommended dosage is once daily for the XE formulation.

The following month, the patient went to another pharmacy to have her prescription filled. The prescription was therefore transferred with the remaining 12 refills. Assuming that the information initially entered into the computer was correct, the pharmacist perpetuated the error by transferring Timoptic XE 0.5%. The patient therefore used the incorrect drug for a full year until all the refills were exhausted, at which time the prescriber was called for verbal authority to refill the prescription. When contacted, the ophthalmologist indicated that he did not prescribe Timoptic XE 0.5% initially. In addition, he explained that he would not pre-scribe Timoptic XE 0.5% with a twice-daily dosing schedule. The pharmacist there-fore contacted the original pharmacy and asked that the original prescription be retrieved. It was at this point that the error was detected. Fortunately, the patient suffered no long-term effects.

Possible Contributory Factors

- The similarities between Timoptic 0.5% and Timoptic XE 0.5% increase the likelihood of selecting the incorrect drug when scrolling through drug names in the computer.
- The technician filled the prescription by reading the computer-generated hard copy.
- The pharmacist and technician did not make full use of the patient history.
- Both the transferring and receiving pharmacists failed to check the dosage for appropriateness.

Preventive Strategies for Transferred Prescriptions

- In accepting prescription transfers, repeat the information as understood by you to the transferring pharmacist.
- If possible, ask that the information be faxed.
- Carefully check the information for appropriateness.
- Consider requesting that a copy of the original prescription be faxed for your records.

Drug Stability and Storage

Most medications dispensed by pharmacists are stored at room temperature and, if stored appropriately, are stable up to the date of expiry on the product. However, many pharmacists may be unaware of the specific storage require-ment and limited stability of some products.

Case 5.13

Clavulin-200 suspension
Sig: i tsp bid
Dispense: 10 days

This prescription, for a 3-year-old child, was given to a pharmacy technician for processing. It was determined that a total volume of 100 mL was required to fill the prescription. As a result, two 70-mL bottles (a total volume of 140 mL) of the recon-stituted suspension of Clavulin-200 was dispensed. The pharmacist checked the prescription and dispensed the medication with appropriate patient counseling.

Five days later, the child's mother noticed the printed information on the product label which stated that the "reconstituted suspension is stable for 7 days under refrigeration." She therefore returned to the pharmacy and questioned why she was given a 10-day supply of a medication that is stable for only 7 days. The pharmacist apologized for the error and provided her with another 70 mL bottle of reconstituted Clavulin-200 suspension.

Preventive Strategies for Drug Stability and Storage

- Ensure that all pharmacy staff are aware of the many drugs which require specific storage conditions and limited stability.
- Keep and post an updated list of these products as a quick reference (see Table 5.1).
- Consider the stability of a product in determining the quantity to be dispensed.
- Consider the implications of dispensing less than the full package size of drugs with limited stability, such as Flamazine cream and Elidel cream.
- In counseling the patient or agent, include storage and stability information. This is especially critical when one of the products listed in Table 5.1 is being dispensed.

TABLE 5.1
Storage and Stability Requirements

Product	Storage Requirement	Stability
Andriol Capsules	Pharmacist to store in refrigerator between 2°C and 8°C; patient must store between 15°C and 25°C.	Patient must use within 90 days.
Benzamycin Topical Gel	Mixed formulation should be stored under refrigeration (between 2°C and 8°C).	To be used within 3 months of dispensing.
Benzaclin Topical Gel	Mixed formulation should be stored between 15°C and 25°C.	To be used within 2 months after mixing by pharmacist.
Biaxin Oral Suspension	Reconstituted suspension must not be refrigerated.	Reconstituted suspension should be discarded after 14 days.
Capex Shampoo	To be stored at room temperature between 15°C and 30°C.	To be discarded 3 months after mixing date.
Clavulin-200 Clavulin-400	Reconstituted suspension to be refrigerated.	Reconstituted suspension is stable for 7 days under refrigeration.

(continued)

TABLE 5.1
Storage and Stability Requirements (Continued)

Product	Storage Requirement	Stability
Clindoxyl Gel	Pharmacist to store in refrigerator between 2°C and 8°C; patient must store between 15°C and 25°C.	Patient to discard after 120 days.
Elidel Cream	Store between 15°C and 30°C.	Contents should be used within 12 weeks after opening.
Estalis/Estalis Sequi	Pharmacist to store in refrigerator between 2°C and 8°C; patient may store patches between 20°C and 25°C	Patient should use patches within 6 months or before expiry date on the package.
Flamazine Cream	Store at 8°C to 25°C.	Tubes to be discarded 7 days after opening; 500-g jars to be discarded 24 hours after opening.
Fucithalmic Viscous Eyedrops	Store at 2°C to 25°C.	To be discarded 1 month after opening.
Miacalcin NS	Pharmacist to store in refrigerator between 2°C and 8°C; patient should store at room temperature below 25°C.	Patient must use within 4 weeks.
Ventolin Respirator Solution	Store below 25°C.	Discard within 1 month after opening.
Xalatan ophthalmic solution	Once opened, store bottle at room temperature up to 25°C.	Discard 6 weeks after opening.
Xalacom ophthalmic solution	Once opened, store bottle at room temperature up to 25°C.	Discard 10 weeks after opening.

Note: This is not an exhaustive list. This list should be updated on a regular basis.
Source: Compendium of Pharmaceuticals and Specialties. Ottawa: Canadian Pharmacists Association; 2004.

MANUFACTURER ISSUES

Manufacturers are key stakeholders in the prevention of medication incidents. Confusing drug names, packaging, labeling, and drug codes have all contributed to medication incidents.

Look-Alike Packaging

Pharmaceutical manufacturers usually design their labels to be recognized across their product lines. In addition, containers of the same size, shape, and color are often used. The result is look-alike packaging for different products. Although Cases 5.14 and 5.15 occurred in Canada, look-alike packaging is a challenging issue in all pharmacy practice sites.

Case 5.14

A prescription for Engerix B for a 6-year-old was presented to a technician for filling. The prescription was entered into the computer correctly. However, a second technician selected Engerix B adult (1 mL) to be dispensed. The pharmacist checked the prescription, including the drug identification number (DIN), but did not detect the error. Fortunately, the error was detected by the physician prior to administration.

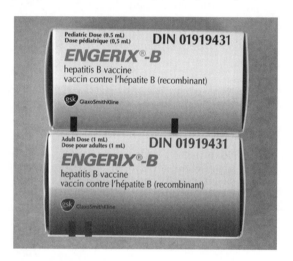

Possible Contributory Factors

- Both products come in packages of identical size and shape.

- Health Canada's Therapeutic Products Directorate will assign a single DIN for products of varying sizes provided that all other product characteristics, including product name, manufacturer's name, dosage form, route of administration, medicinal ingredient(s), and corresponding strength(s), are identical. Since only the volume differs between the Engerix products, they both have identical DINs. Other products that share the same DIN but have different volumes can be found in Table 5.2.

- The technician affixed the computer-generated label to the product, thereby obscuring the "Adult Dose" designation on the product packaging.

- The adult dose is most often dispensed and may have influenced the selection of the incorrect product.

Case 5.15

A community pharmacy ordered three vials of dexamethasone injection 4 mg/mL. After receiving the product, the pharmacy technician placed the three vials in the storage location designated for cyanocobalamin injection 1,000 μg/mL because of the look-alike packaging.

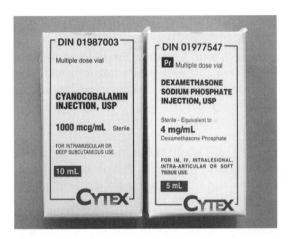

Some time later, a patient requested a vial of "vitamin B$_{12}$ injection." The pharmacist proceeded to the storage location of cyanocobalamin injection and retrieved a vial of dexamethasone injection previously placed there in error. Fortunately the error was detected before the patient left the pharmacy. Had the patient left the pharmacy before the error was found, there would have been no personal information available to contact the patient, since a prescription is not required for the sale of cyanocobalamin injection in Canada, although such a prescription is required in the United States.

Possible Contributory Factors

- The packages of both products are similar in size, shape, and color.

- The labeling is similar in appearance.

- The pharmacy technician was familiar with the packaging of cyanocobalamin injection. Therefore, on receiving the dexamethasone injection, she likely glanced at the label and assumed that it was cyanocobalamin injection. Studies have shown that we often "see" what is familiar rather than what is actually there.

- Verification of the DIN is a key step in the dispensing process to ensure that the correct drug is being dispensed. However, since the sale of cyanocobalamin does not require a prescription in Canada, this process did not take place.

Preventive Strategies for Look-Alike Packaging

- Use extra caution in dispensing products with similar packaging and DIN or NDC numbers.
- Double-check the inventory to confirm that the right drug is in the right storage location.
- Consider purchasing a different brand of one of the products to reduce the potential of a mixup.
- Check all digits of the DIN or NDC number of the product being dispensed.
- Consider the patient's age and weight to assess the appropriateness of the medication.
- Teach pharmacy staff to avoid placing the computer-generated label on the product in a manner that obscures important information.
- Contact your software provider to discuss possible built-in alerts to detect the presence of identical DINs in different drug files.
- Manufacturers must take steps to ensure that packaging, labeling, and product appearance are distinct and clearly identify different products.
- Educate all pharmacy staff about the issue of identical DINs and the potential for error. See Table 5.2 for a partial list of these products.
- Consider storing these and other similar products in separate locations.
- Although the DIN assigned to both Engerix products is identical, the assigned bar code is unique to each product. The use of bar-code technology during the dispensing process can therefore reduce the potential for error. Consider an investment in bar-code technology such as bar-code scanners to confirm that the correct drug is being dispensed.

TABLE 5.2
Products with Identical DINs

Products	DIN
Engerix-B Pediatric Dose Engerix-B Adult Dose	01919431
Fragmin 5000 IU/0.2 mL Fragmin 7500 IU/0.3 mL Fragmin 10000 IU/0.4 mL Fragmin 12500 IU/0.5 mL Fragmin 15000 IU/0.6 mL Fragmin 18000 IU/0.72 mL	02132648
Lovenox 40 mg/0.4 mL Lovenox 60 mg/0.6 mL Lovenox 80 mg/0.8 mL Lovenox 100 mg/1 mL	02236883
Lovenox HP 120 mg/0.8 mL Lovenox HP 150 mg/1 mL	02242692

Suffixes and Line Extensions

Pharmaceutical manufacturers invest significantly in the development of trademarks. An effective brand name can[5]:

- Distinguish a company's product from a competitor's product
- Convey an impression of product quality or another desirable feature
- Generate brand loyalty
- Imply an association with a market leader

With the development of a successful brand name, manufacturers often add additional products to the product line in an effort to capitalize on the many benefits.

Pharmaceutical manufacturers use a variety of terms in describing formulations in which the release of the drug has been modified. These terms include "long acting," "sustained action," "extended release," "sustained release," "modified release," "controlled release," and "controlled delivery." As a result, a variety of suffixes are used in naming these products. Examples include Entex LA, Reminyl ER, Effexor XR, Biaxin XL, Tiazac XC, Isoptin SR, Tegretol CR, Cardizem CD, and (available in Canada) Diamicron MR. In some instances, such as the brand name Unidet, no suffix is used. This lack of consistency can be potentially confusing and may be a contributing factor in medication errors, as illustrated in Cases 5.16 and 5.17.

Case 5.16

This prescription was written by a physician for an 80-year-old patient. The brand name Unidet is no longer used, as the manufacturer has changed the name to Detrol LA. Unlike Detrol LA, Unidet did not have a suffix. As a result, the dispensing pharmacist was not aware that Unidet was the extended-release formulation of tolterodine L-tartrate. The pharmacist therefore substituted Detrol for Detrol LA. The patient took Detrol for a full year until her next visit to the doctor. Upon reviewing the patient's medication, the physician discovered the error.

Possible Contributory Factors

- The name Unidet did not include a suffix indicating that it was an extended-release product.

- The physician wrote Unidet instead of using the current brand name, Detrol LA. The pharmacist was therefore required to make an appropriate substitution.

- Both Detrol and Detrol LA are available in the 2-mg strength.

Case 5.17

A 21-year-old patient presented the prescription shown here to a pharmacist for filling. The pharmacist read the prescription as Tri-cyclen and completed all steps involved in the processing of the prescription. The package was then placed in a drawer for pickup.

The following day, the patient returned to pick up her medication. On this occasion, a second pharmacist retrieved the prescription bag and reviewed the prescription in order to counsel the patient, thus finding that the prescription was actually written for Tri-cyclen Lo, not Tri-cyclen. The correction was, therefore, made.

Preventive Strategies for Suffixes and Line Extensions

- Ensure that all staff are aware of changes in drug names.
- When you are required to make a substitution, always consult an appropriate reference or contact your drug information center to confirm that the correct decision has been made.
- In retrieving stock bottles from storage, always read the original prescription, then compare the product selected to that on the computer-generated hard copy.
- Whenever possible, at least two individuals should be involved in the dispensing of all prescriptions. This provides a key double-check opportunity.

- In dispensing medications, always check the dosing interval for appropriateness.
- Pharmaceutical manufacturers should be encouraged to take steps to improve labeling, packaging, and naming of pharmaceuticals to reduce the risk of incidents.
- Be aware of potentially problematic line extensions that may lead to medication errors (see Table 5.3).

TABLE 5.3
Problematic Line Extensions

Alphagan	Alphagan P
Anaprox	Anaprox DS
Biaxin	Biaxin XL
Cipro	Cipro XL
Dimetane Expectorant C	Dimetane Expectorant DC
Fucidin	Fucidin H
Herplex	Herplex D
Hycomine	Hycomine S
Maxalt	Maxalt RPD
Medrol	Neo-Medrol
Prevex	Prevex B, Prevex HC
Reminyl	Reminyl ER
Stievamycin	Stievamycin Mild, Stievamycin Forte
Tiazac	Tiazac XC
Timoptic	Timoptic XE
Tri-cyclen	Tri-cyclen Lo

RECONCILIATION

Reconciliation ensures that patients receive continuous, uninterrupted care as they move from one part of the health care system to another. However, many patients are at risk of experiencing an adverse drug event as they move between community-based and hospital-based care.

A recent study[6] found that approximately one-quarter of patients discharged from hospital experienced an adverse event, with adverse drug events being the most common. Half of the patients experienced an adverse event that was either preventable or ameliorable.

Effective communication between health care providers in the hospital and community setting is critical to ensure patient safety. Unfortunately this communication is often lacking.

Many community-based pharmacists are aware of the scenario in which a patient presents a written prescription with several prescribed medications and states that he had been discharged from the hospital following a heart attack. The patient then questions whether he should continue to take the medications prescribed prior to hospitalization. The pharmacist's attempt to identify and contact the prescriber to confirm his or her intent is often time-consuming and frequently unsuccessful. At best, patient care is delayed.

A complicating factor can be the therapeutic interchange policy of many hospitals. Following established guidelines, hospital staff can interchange a prescribed drug with another drug of the same therapeutic class as listed in the hospital formulary. For example, a patient who had been taking Zestril can be switched to Altace following admission to the hospital. On being discharged from the hospital, the patient can be at risk of experiencing an adverse drug event unless there is sharing of information between the hospital pharmacist and the community pharmacist providing care to the patient, as shown in Case 5.18.

Case 5.18

A patient taking quinapril was admitted to hospital. Following admission, the hospital therapeutic interchange policy dictated that the patient be switched to ramipril. The patient was later transferred to another hospital and the nurse wrote down the medication orders from the transfer sheet. In error, both quinapril and ramipril were recorded. Fortunately the pharmacist receiving the order questioned the need for both agents and, upon investigation, the error was detected.

Clearly effective communication and the sharing of information must take place between health care providers in various settings. Following a patient's admission to hospital and on discharge from hospital, his or her drug regimen must be part of the discussion between the hospital and the community-based pharmacist. Without it, patient safety will be compromised.

In the United States, the Joint Commission on Accreditation of Healthcare Organizations (JCAHO) has required the reconciliation of medications from admission to discharge to the next level of care.

PHARMACY WORKLOAD

Work overload is one issue that pharmacists often point to as a reason for medication incidents. Pharmacists in both hospital and community settings rank work overload as the most significant cause of dispensing errors.[7] The potential for error is compounded by the stress experienced by the pharmacist who has a maximum time allowance to dispense prescriptions.

However, there has been much debate regarding the relationship of work-load to dispensing errors. One study compared workload and error rates and found no association between work volume and the number of dispensing errors.[8] In another study that looked at error rates at low- (less than 900 pre-scriptions per week), medium- (900 – 1,400 prescriptions per week), and high-volume (over 1,400 prescriptions per week) retail outlets, Anthony Grasha[9] found that more "misfills" were associated with the low-volume stores. He suggests that with less work to do, boredom may occur, and it becomes easier to focus on nontask issues that interfere with performance. He also found that shifting from high- to low-workload conditions was more detrimental for pharmacists working in high-volume stores. They made more process errors when workload dropped than they did while maintaining a fast pace. However, when workload increased in the low-volume stores, pharma-cists made fewer errors. Working at a relatively faster pace seemed to increase task engagement and concentration, and this resulted in fewer mistakes. Grasha points out that none of this is justification to encourage long workdays or higher rates of dispensing medications. Like everyone else, pharmacists have different thresholds for workload and how much they can do safely without burning out.

He also adds that we cannot generalize about how detrimental any given factor will be in the dispensing process. The dispensing process is multifaceted and subject to influences that may not work across the board in ways that con-ventional wisdom suggests they should.

Preventive Strategies Relating to Pharmacy Workload

- Consider the implications of establishing minimum prescription filling rates and a maximum allowable time for filling of a prescription.
- Consider staffing needs based on the volume of prescriptions filled.
- Make sure that support staff is adequately trained to handle all nonprofes-sional activities, thereby reducing the pharmacist's workload.
- Include appropriate breaks during the pharmacist's shift.
- Avoid dramatic shifts in workload by finding ways to better distribute tasks.

ENVIRONMENT

A number of studies have examined the relationship between the environment and medication incident rates. Factors examined include interruptions and dis-tractions, lighting, noise, and temperature.

One study, which took place in an ambulatory pharmacy, demonstrated a relationship between interruptions and distractions with dispensing error rates.[10] The error rate for the filling of prescriptions during which there were one or more distractions was 6.55%, compared with an error rate of 5.64% for prescriptions for which there were no distractions.

Another study demonstrated the relationship between the level of lighting and the prescription dispensing error rate in a high-volume outpatient pharmacy.

An illumination level of 146 footcandles was associated with a significantly lower error rate (2.6%) than the baseline level of 45 footcandles (3.8%).[11] However, Caverly[12] suggests that there is no single easy answer to appropriate lighting levels. Not only does it take different lighting levels to perform different tasks (data entry, product location, counting, and verification), but too much lighting can be as bad as too little. Excessive lighting levels produce glare, troublesome reflections, deep shadows, and excessive contrasts. The result: headaches and fatigue, with lower productivity and increased errors.

Noise has also been identified as a factor that may affect performance. Glass and Singer[13] suggest that uncontrollable and unpredictable noises (such as paging, telephone rings, printers, faxes, and conversation) might be associated with an increased frequency of dispensing errors, as seen in Case 5.19.

Case 5.19

While checking a prescription written for Vasotec 10 mg, the pharmacist was interrupted by a telephone call. The pharmacist continued to perform this critical checking process while communicating with a patient on the telephone. As a result, he did not notice that the technician had inadvertently selected the Zocor 10 mg stock bottle to fill the prescription. The patient therefore received Zocor 10 mg instead of Vasotec 10 mg. Fortunately, the patient had previously been taking Vasotec and therefore detected the error before consuming the wrong drug.

Possible Contributory Factors

- The pharmacist was interrupted during the checking process.
- The pharmacist attempted to complete two different tasks simultaneously, with both requiring his full attention.
- The stock bottles of Vasotec 10 mg and Zocor 10 mg are similar in size, shape, and color.
- The technician selected Zocor 10 mg in error because it was inadvertently stored with the Vasotec 10 mg.

Preventive Strategies Related to Environment

- Assess the work environment for appropriate lighting, temperature control, noise level, distractions, clutter, and the performance of unrelated tasks.
- Remove all activities and items that may be potentially distracting (e.g., the employee time clock).
- Consider investing in Interactive Voice Response (IVR) technology, thereby reducing the number of telephone calls into the dispensary.
- Determine whether the pharmacy has an efficient and effective environment—a proper storage area with adequate space, that labels face forward,

that there is no clutter and sufficient space for work (counter and walking area) and for storage.[3]

- In the dispensary, use the "sterile cockpit" concept for pilots, so that conversations not related to dispensing are not permitted during critical functions (for pilots, the cutoff point for non-work-related conversation is anything below 10,000 feet). In addition, each of the pharmacy's functions must be clearly defined as to procedures for performing it, including who will do it, where it is done, and when it is done.
- Telephones should be placed where they are convenient but not too distracting.
- Work areas should be designed for smooth work flow from one task to the next.
- Avoid performing multiple tasks during the prescription checking process.
- Educate the staff to avoid interrupting the pharmacist while he or she is checking a prescription.
- The pharmacy support staff should screen incoming calls, thereby eliminating unnecessary interruptions.
- Pharmacy technicians should be trained to handle as many issues as possible, thereby reducing the pharmacist's workload.
- Whenever possible, use a designated pharmacist for troubleshooting, so that the dispensing pharmacist can concentrate solely on the dispensing of prescriptions.

ORGANIZATIONAL ISSUES

Organizational failures can also contribute to medication incidents. Large organizations possess complex systems that are multilayered, involving multiple stakeholders. Health care providers perform exacting tasks under considerable time pressures.

Management must therefore take steps to effectively manage obstacles inherent in complex organizations in order to achieve an environment of patient safety. These steps may include the following:

- Establish a culture of patient safety. Error reduction must be an explicit organizational goal. Each member of the health care team must make patient safety a daily commitment and focus.
- Drug information references must be current and available to health care providers when and where they need them in a readily usable format. In one study, lack of knowledge about drugs and lack of information about patients were the two most common system failures, accounting for 40% of injury-producing errors.[14]
- If a medication error or near miss does occur at your practice site, analyze the incident to determine possible contributory factors, develop a list of recommendations to prevent a recurrence, and share the information with all pharmacy staff. The ASSESS-ERR tool from the Institute for Safe Medication Practices (ISMP) (available at www.ismp.org/Tools/AssessERR.pdf) can be used to assist in analyzing the incident.

- Learn from incidents that have occurred at other practice sites through the ISMP Medication Safety Alert, the ISMP Canada Safety Bulletin, and other published accounts of medication errors. A list of Web sites is provided in Table 5.4.
- Implement prevention strategies to ensure that similar incidents will not occur in your practice.
- Share information, as this is also an important step. Information regarding medication incidents and prevention strategies must be shared among health care providers, between departments, and with other health care institutions.
- Health care providers should be encouraged to report medication incidents without fear of punishment or assignment of blame. The blaming of individuals is a dominant tradition. Therefore, organizations may impose overt or covert sanctions against individuals who make mistakes. The resulting fear of punishment discourages reporting and discussing medication incidents.
- Incidents of medication errors can be reported to ISMP and ISMP Canada.
- Assess staffing and scheduling policies for effectiveness. Ensure appropriate staffing levels to meet work demands throughout the day. Excessively long shifts without breaks can cause fatigue, which can be a contributing factor to medication incidents.
- All staff must be appropriately trained in order to fulfill their required duties in a safe manner. Staff should undertake only those duties for which they are appropriately trained and that they are qualified to perform.

TABLE 5.4
Useful Web Site Resources

Resource	Website
The Institute for Safe Medication Practices	www.ismp.org
Joint Commission on Accreditation of Healthcare Organizations	www.jcaho.org/
Massachusetts Coalition for the Prevention of Medical Errors	www.macoalition.org/
U.S. Food and Drug Administration	www.fda.gov/
The Institute for Safe Medication Practices Canada	www.ismp-canada.org/
National Coordinating Council for Medication Error	www.nccmerp.org/
Reporting and Prevention Medical Error Recognition and Revision Strategies	www.med-errs.com/

SUMMARY

In this chapter some of the underlying root causes of medication error are discussed. The root cause of medication error is often a result of system failure and a breakdown in the dispensing process.

Humans are fallible and likely to make errors. Therefore, defenses must be built within the system to prevent or reduce the likelihood of an error occurring. Errors in specialty practices are discussed in Chapter 6.

Reflective Questions

1. Identify a specific example in your practice of confirmation bias that has led to a medication incident. Discuss prevention strategies for this incident.
2. Identify an incident that has occurred during the dispensing process. Discuss prevention strategies for this incident.
3. Identify products with similar packaging in your practice site. Discuss ways of reducing the likelihood that a medication incident will occur.
4. Develop a list of medications containing suffixes and line extensions that may be problematic in your practice; be sure to include nonprescription medications if appropriate.
5. Assess your current work environment in the areas of noise level, lighting level, and distractions/interruptions. Identify areas that could be improved in order to reduce the chance that a medication incident will occur.

REFERENCES

1. Grasha AF, O'Neill MO. Cognitive processess in medication errors. *US Pharm*, 1996;21:96–109.
2. Leape L. A systems analysis approach to medical error. In: Cohen M, ed. *Medication Errors: Causes, Prevention, and Risk Management*. Boston: Jones and Bartlett; 2000:2.1–2.10.
3. Cohen M. Preventing dispensing error. In: Cohen M, ed. *Medication Errors: Causes, Prevention, and Risk Management*. Boston: Jones and Bartlett; 2000:9.1–9.19.
4. Compendium of Pharmaceuticals and Specialties. Ottawa: Canadian Pharmacists Association; 2004;794:1060.
5. Cohen M. The role of pharmaceutical trademarks in mediation errors. In: Cohen M, ed. *Medication Errors: Causes, Prevention, and Risk Management*. Boston: Jones and Bartlett; 2000:12.8.
6. Forster AJ, Clark HD, Menard A, et al. Adverse events among medical patients after discharge from hospital. *CMAJ*. 2004;170(3):345–349.
7. Davis NM, Cohen MR. Ten steps for ensuring dispensary accuracy. *Am Pharm*. 1994;NS34(7):22–23.
8. Kistner UA, Keith MR, Sergeant KA, et al. Accuracy of dispensing in a high-volume, hospital based outpatient pharmacy. *Am J Hosp Pharm*. 1994;51:2793–2797.

9. Grasha AF. Misconceptions about pharmacy workload. *Can Pharm J.* 2001;134(3): 26–25.
10. Flynn EA, Barker KN, Gibson JT, et al. Impact of interruptions and distractions on dispensing errors in an ambulatory care pharmacy. *Am J Health-Syst Pharm.* 1999;56:1319–1325.
11. Buchanan TL, Barker KN, Gibson JT, et al. Illumination and errors in dispensing. *Am J Hosp Pharm.* 1991;48:2137–2145.
12. Caverly WM. Improving efficiencies and reducing medication errors. *Effic Pharm.* 2000;3(2):2.
13. Glass DC, Singer JE. Experimental studies of uncontrollable and unpredictable noise. *Rep Res Psychol.* 1973;4:165–183.
14. Leape LL, Bates DW, Cullen DJ, et al. Systems analysis of adverse drug events. *JAMA.* 1995:274:35–43.

Chapter 6

Causes and Preventive Strategies in Specialty Practices

Objective

After completing this chapter, the reader will be able to:

- Identify various types of medication incidents frequently seen in specialty practices
- Recognize similar situations in pharmacy practice that could lead to medication incidents
- Identify preventive strategies for incidents that may occur in specialty practices
- Apply the knowledge gained to your current practice with a view to preventing future incidents
- Recognize the many factors that affect the stability of extemporaneous products
- Identify factors that place pediatric patients at increase risk of experiencing an adverse event

Although medication discrepancies and incidents can occur in any area of pharmacy practice, there are some types of specialty practices where there is a particularly high risk of incidents or where incidents can be more serious, even fatal. This chapter focuses on incidents involving pediatrics, compounding, nonprescription medications, immunization, and methadone.

PEDIATRICS

Pediatric patients are at increased risk for experiencing a medication incident. A study by Harvard Medical School found that children are three times as likely as adults to get the wrong dose of a drug.[1] As a result of immature body organs and increased sensitivity to the effects of drugs, pediatric patients are especially at risk for increased morbidity and mortality. Other factors that place pediatric patients at increased risk of experiencing an adverse drug event include the following[2]:

- Different and changing pharmacokinetic parameters between patients at various ages and stages of maturity.
- The need for calculation of individualized doses based on the patient's age, weight (mg/kg), body surface area (mg/m^2), and clinical condition.
- A lack of available dosage forms and concentrations appropriate for administration to neonates, infants, and children. Frequently, dosage formulations are extemporaneously compounded and information regarding stability, compatibility, and bioavailability is sometimes lacking.
- The need for precise dose measurement and appropriate drug delivery systems.
- A lack of published information or approved labeling regarding dosing, pharmacokinetics, safety, efficacy, and clinical use of drugs in the pediatric population.

Pharmacists and pharmacy technicians often receive prescriptions with vague instructions such as, "Take as directed." In some cases, the patients have been given the specific instructions in written form for easy reference. However, often the patient "did not hear" or cannot recall the verbal instructions given. The potential for error also exists when the instructions given to the patient or parent are not the same as those written on the prescription, as seen in Case 6.1.

Case 6.2 and Case 6.3 highlight the need to double-check the prescribed dose for appropriateness based on the child's age and weight.

Case 6.1

A 15-year-old boy was seen by a pediatrician at a neurology clinic and was given the following prescription.

Topamax 100 mg twice daily
Dispense: 2 months

The child's mother was also given the printed instruction sheet shown in Table 6.1.

TABLE 6.1
Printed Instruction Sheet

Date	Medication	Morning Dose	Evening Dose
September 4, 2002	Topamax		50 mg
September 9, 2002		50 mg	50 mg
September 14, 2002		50 mg	75 mg
September 19, 2002		75 mg	75 mg
September 24, 2002		75 mg	100 mg
September 29, 2002		100 mg	100 mg

Assuming that the 25-mg tablet would be dispensed, the pediatrician verbally instructed the mother to give her son two tablets each night for 5 days, then two tablets twice daily for 5 days, etc.

Later in the day, the child's father presented the prescription to the local community pharmacy for filling. Unaware of the detailed instruction sheet, the pharmacist dispensed the 100-mg tablet with the label instruction to give one tablet twice daily.

Without reading the label on the prescription vial, the mother gave the child two tablets, which resulted in an initial dosage of 200 mg or four times the intended dose.

The following morning, the child was observed to be drowsy and disoriented. The mother then checked the contents of the prescription vial and called the pharmacist to report that an error had been made.

Possible Contributory Factors

- The instructions given to the mother by the prescriber were different from those written on the prescription.

- The pharmacist was not given the detailed instruction sheet and therefore was unaware of its existence.

- The physician assumed that the 25-mg tablets would be dispensed.

- The pharmacist did not question the relatively high initial dose of 100 mg twice daily. He was likely unaware of the manufacturer's recommendation that therapy be initiated at a lower dose, followed by titration as needed and tolerated to an effective dose.

- The child's father presented the prescription for filling. The child's mother might have detected the error while being counseled by the pharmacist, since she had taken the child to the doctor.

- The child's mother did not read the prescription label before giving the medication.

- Patients often use more than one pharmacy. Therefore the pharmacist may have thought that the patient had previously received the titrating dose from another pharmacy or mail order.

Case 6.2

A father took the following prescription for his 5-year-old son to his local pharmacy for filling.

Chloroquine Phosphate
100 mg once weekly for 6 weeks,
starting 1 week prior to trip

The father explained that his family, along with his brother's family, would be traveling to the Dominican Republic for a winter vacation and therefore required the chloroquine phosphate for malaria prophylaxis.

The pharmacy technician prepared a suspension of chloroquine phosphate with the final concentration of 15 mg/mL. The label instructions therefore read to "Give 6.7 mL (100 mg) once weekly for 6 weeks, starting 1 week prior to trip."

The pharmacist provided appropriate counseling. However, the father questioned the accuracy of the dose. He indicated that his nephew, who is of the same age as his son, was given a dosage of 10 mL weekly.

The pharmacist therefore doubled-checked the prescription and the calculation used in compounding the suspension. Using a dosing guideline of 5 mg/kg chloroquine base once weekly[3] and the child's weight (determined to be 20 kg), the pharmacist confirmed that the recommended dose would be 100 mg chloroquine *base* once weekly. A call to the prescriber confirmed that the intended dose was 100 mg chloroquine base once weekly and not 100 mg chloroquine phosphate.

Since Novo-Chloroquine 250-mg tablets (155 mg chloroquine base per tablet) were used in preparing the oral suspension, the label instructions were corrected to "Give 10.8 mL once weekly for 6 weeks, starting 1 week prior to trip."

Possible Contributory Factors

- The prescriber did not specify chloroquine base on the prescription.
- The child's weight was not included on the prescription.
- The pharmacist did not initially inquire about the child's weight and therefore could not confirm the accuracy of the prescribed dose.
- The pharmacist's lack of knowledge of the difference between chloroquine phosphate and the chloroquine base.
- The product label of chloroquine phosphate did not clearly show the relationship between chloroquine phosphate and the chloroquine base.

Case 6.3

An 11-year-old boy was seen at the outpatient clinic of the local hospital and received the prescription shown here for the relief of pain. The prescription was taken to a nearby pharmacy for processing.

A pharmacy technician entered the prescription into the computer and a second technician prepared and labeled 50 mL of the codeine syrup for checking by the pharmacist. On checking the prescription, the pharmacist noticed that despite a dosage of 20 to 30 mL every 4 hours, only 50 mL of codeine syrup was being dispensed. The prescribed dose was therefore checked for appropriateness. The pharmacist identified that based on a concentration of 5 mg codeine per mL, the prescribed dose would be equivalent to 100 to 150 mg. Assuming five doses per day, the total daily dosage would be 500 to 750 mg codeine per day—a potentially lethal dose.

A call to the prescribing physician at the hospital confirmed that he intended to prescribe 20 to 30 mg or 4 to 6 mL codeine per dose and not 20 to 30 mL. The correction was made and the appropriate dose given.

Possible Contributory Factors

- The erroneous interchanging of "mg" and "mL" is often seen in pharmacy practice. Since dosages of oral liquids are most often written as "mL," in this instance the prescribing physician likely wrote what was most familiar.

- Both the pharmacy technician who entered the prescription into the computer and the technician who prepared the codeine syrup failed to detect the relationship between the dose of 20 to 30 mL and the total prescribed volume of only 50 mL.

Preventive Strategies for Pediatrics

- Prescribers should be encouraged to indicate, on the prescription, the weight of the child, the calculated dose, and the dose equation (the mg/kg basis of the dose). The pharmacist should verify the mg/kg dose and double check the calculation to confirm that the appropriate dose has been prescribed.
- Always ensure that the patient/agent is aware of the dose to be taken/given. This is especially important when the prescriber writes vague instructions such as "Take as directed." Ask the patient/agent, "How did the doctor tell you to take/give this medication?"
- Provide an appropriate measuring device when you are dispensing liquids. Place a mark on the device to clearly identify the volume of liquid to be administered to the child.
- Have readily available and consult appropriate, up-to-date drug references whenever the pharmacist is not familiar with the appropriate dosing of a drug. This is especially critical in dispensing medication for the pediatric population.
- Whenever possible, a second individual should perform an independent check of all calculations without prior knowledge of the results of the first calculation.
- In dispensing oral liquids, be alert for the potential interchanging of "mg" and "mL."
- Provide the child's parent or caregiver with both verbal and written information regarding the medication and side effects that may be experienced. He or she should be encouraged to report any unexpected side effects.
- Ensure that all staff are appropriately trained in preparing and dispensing drugs to the pediatric population.
- Contact your software vendor to set weight-based dosage limits in the computer system, thereby alerting staff to potential excessive dosages.

- Pharmacy technicians should play a key role in identifying and preventing potential medication errors. Educate and train all pharmacy staff on fulfilling this critical role. A key component of the plan should be the review and discussion of potential medication errors and actual errors that occurred at various pharmacies. This would greatly reduce the possibility of the same error occurring at your pharmacy.

COMPOUNDING

Although most prescriptions are for medications provided by pharmaceutical manufacturers, the pharmacist or pharmacy technician is often required to prepare a number of extemporaneous compounds for a variety of situations. As previously mentioned, pediatric patients require unique dosages not commercially available; therefore these must be prepared by the pharmacist.

Pharmacists and pharmacy technicians must possess the required specialized knowledge and skill to prepare extemporaneous preparations accurately and safely. Appropriate policies, standards, and procedures must be strictly adhered to in order to prevent medication incidents, as seen in Cases 6.4, 6.5, and 6.6.

Case 6.4

A pharmacy technician, in the process of setting up a batch preparation of dialysis solution, picked up a carton of 12 × 250 mL concentrated potassium chloride 2 mmol/mL bottles, instead of a carton of 12 × 250 mL bottles of 23.4% sodium chloride (NaCl) for injection (see Figs. 6.1 and 6.2).

Since 85 mL of sodium chloride solution was needed for each 3-L dialysis solution and because one batch preparation was 35 bags, an entire carton of 12 bottles of 250 mL NaCl solution was required. The cartons of stock potassium chloride solutions were located near the sodium chloride solutions.

During the preparation process, 85 mL of potassium chloride 2 mEq/mL (2 mmol/mL) was added to the 3-L bags of dialysis solution. Each of the 3-L solutions contained a total of 170 mmol potassium chloride. This amount, given over a short period of time, such as 3 hours, is lethal.

When one of the renal dialysis patients died suddenly, the physician identified a serum potassium of almost 8 mmol/L. An immediate laboratory test carried out on the dialysis solution revealed the error. The hospital then recalled the remaining bags of dialysis solution.

Officials reviewed the charts of all other patients who had received continuous dialysis since the batch had been produced. It was determined that a second patient was probably exposed to this same batch and had died as a result of hyperkalemia. Five of the dialysis bags had been utilized for two patients and the other 30 bags were successfully retrieved from the patient care area.

Note: This case is adapted with permission from ISMP Canada. Concentrated potassium chloride: a recurring danger. ISMP Can Saf Bull 2004;4(3):1–2.

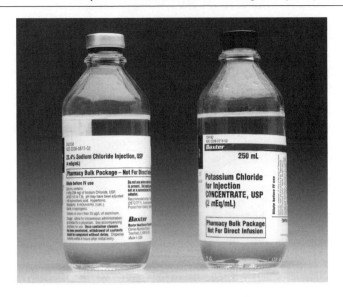

FIGURE 6.1 Bottles of sodium chloride injection (left) and potassium chloride injection (right). (Photo courtesy of ISMP Canada.)

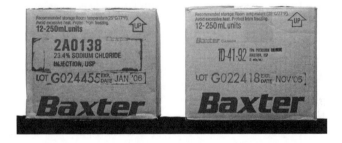

FIGURE 6.2 Bottles of sodium chloride injection (left) and potassium chloride injection (right). (Photo courtesy of ISMP Canada.)

Case 6.5

Many pediatric antibiotics are sold to pharmacies in a powdered form to be reconstituted with water just prior to being dispensed.

There have been a number of reports of the incorrect volume of water being added to the drug powder, thereby resulting in an incorrect concentration of drug being dispensed.

A pediatrician prescribed 100 mL of amoxicillin 250 mg/5 mL for a 6-year-old child, with the directions to give 1 teaspoonful three times daily until finished. A technician entered the prescription into the computer as 100 mL Novamoxin 250 mg/5 mL (Mixed Berry flavor). A second technician retrieved the correct bottle from the shelf and read the directions for reconstituting the antibiotic on the bottle. The wording states, "add 60 mL water in two portions. . . ." The technician added two lots of 60 mL water for a total of 120 mL instead of two lots of 30 mL for a total of 60 mL.

This resulted in a total volume of 160 mL instead of the intended 100 mL. The final concentration was approximately 156 mg/5mL instead of the intended 250 mg/5 mL. The child would therefore receive an almost 40% reduction in the intended dose, with potential adverse results.

On checking the prescription, the pharmacist did not detect the error because he had often dispensed 150 mL Novamoxin 250 mg/5mL in the same-size bottle. Fortunately, when counseling the child's parent on the use of the antibiotic for 7 days, the pharmacist noted the relatively large volume of liquid and questioned the technician regarding the volume of water added. The error was therefore detected and a new bottle of the suspension prepared correctly and dispensed to the parent with apologies for the error.

Possible Contributory Factors

- Misinterpretation of the manufacturer's directions for reconstituting the antibiotic.

- The bottles of both the 100-mL and 150-mL Novamoxin 250 mg/5 mL are similar in appearance and identical in size and shape.

- The bottle lacked any line or mark indicating the height of the 100 mL of suspension.

- The technician was a new graduate with little practical experience.

Case 6.6

```
(Kg) _____ (cm)
(Metronidazole)
Flagyl 100mg TID po
90 tablets              Repeat x ___3___
```

The prescription shown here was written for a 2-year-old child and taken to a local pharmacy for processing. Since Flagyl 100-mg tablets are not commercially available, the pharmacist asked a pharmacy technician to prepare an oral suspension of metronidazole.

The technician first crushed the required number of metronidazole 250-mg tablets into a fine powder using a mortar and pestle. A small amount of water was added while stirring to form a smooth paste. Enough simple syrup was then gradually added while stirring to make the final required volume and concentration.

Later that day, the father returned for the medication. While counseling on the medication, the pharmacist explained the need for the product to be kept in the refrigerator. The father then indicated that owing to an extended period of traveling, it would be difficult to refrigerate the medication. On checking various references, the pharmacist could find no data supporting the stability of the prepared product at room temperature for an extended period of time. As a result, the prepared product was discarded and the metronidazole suspension remade using an appropriate formulation that rendered it stable at room temperature for a minimum of 30 days.[4]

Preventive Strategies for Compounding

- Review the process for the preparation and checking of extemporaneous products. Ensure that independent double checks are in place.
- Make sure all staff engaged in extemporaneous preparation are appropriately trained.
- Pharmacists and pharmacy technicians must be familiar with the many factors that affect the stability of extemporaneous preparations.
- Adhere to published formulas for which there are adequate stability data. Other factors affecting the stability of extemporaneous preparations include the vehicle used, drug concentration, preservative used, brand of ingredients, flavoring, presence of excipients, particle size, storage conditions, humidity, temperature, air, and light.[5]
- Consider various published formulas and select the most appropriate.
- In preparing extemporaneous products, clearly document the formula used so that it can be duplicated for future prescription refills.
- Be careful in extrapolating. This is especially important in determining an appropriate expiry date. Ensure that the specific expiry date is affixed to the container. If an ingredient is unavailable, contact your drug information center for guidance.
- The appropriate storage container should be used. Amber glass bottles are usually recommended to enhance stability.
- Store concentrated potassium chloride separately in a secure area.
- Attach auxiliary labels to drugs that have a high potential for causing patient harm, thereby alerting staff.
- Consider purchasing either potassium chloride or sodium chloride from different vendors to avoid packaging similarities.
- Use commercially available solutions whenever possible, thereby avoiding the need for compounding.
- Use premixed, diluted solutions of electrolytes in a standard concentration for IV admixture.
- Educate the patient or agent regarding storage condition and the need to shake all suspensions before administering.
- The manufacturers should consider a change in the wording of the directions for reconstituting antibiotic suspensions. The new wording should clearly articulate that a total of 60 mL of water is to be added in two portions of 30 mL each.
- The bottle for each volume of a suspension should be unique. Or, at a minimum, each bottle should have a clear line or mark indicating 100 mL and 150 mL.
- Consider the patient's travel plans and the possibility of refrigerating the final product.

NONPRESCRIPTION MEDICATIONS

Product labels can be especially confusing to the lay person purchasing a non-prescription drug. The manufacturer's failure to clearly express the product strength can lead to dosing errors, as seen in Cases 6.7 and 6.8.

Case 6.7

Mr. Smith, a 63- year-old patient, was prescribed ferrous sulfate 300 mg to be taken once daily. His wife presented the prescription to the pharmacist, who suggested that the product be bought as a nonprescription item. Mrs. Smith was given a bottle of 100 ferrous sulfate 300-mg tablets with appropriate counseling, including instructions that her husband take one tablet daily. Mrs. Smith observed that the manufacturer's label indicated that each tablet contained 300 mg ferrous sulfate but did not notice that, in much smaller print, each tablet was said to contain 60 mg elemental iron.

Approximately 3 months later, Mrs. Smith returned to the pharmacy to purchase a second bottle of ferrous sulfate 300-mg tablets and was given the same brand. However, she did not notice that the manufacturer had changed the product label to reflect the elemental iron content. The new label therefore indicated that each tablet contained 60 mg of elemental iron and in much smaller print, 300 mg of ferrous sulfate. As before, the patient continued to take one tablet daily.

Following the consumption of approximately two-thirds of the bottle, Mrs. Smith observed the label change and assumed that the pharmacist had given her the incorrect strength. Not wanting to return an almost empty bottle, she decided to give her husband five tablets per dose or 300 mg of elemental iron.

A few days later, Mrs. Smith returned to the pharmacy with the empty bottle and insisted that she be given the correct strength since "I was given the wrong strength the last time." The pharmacist therefore explained the relationship between the elemental iron and ferrous sulfate content.

Possible Contributory Factors

- Like most patients, Mrs. Smith did not understand the relationship between elemental iron and ferrous sulfate.
- Lack of labeling standard. While some manufacturers highlight the elemental iron content, others highlight the ferrous sulfate content.
- No discussion took place between the pharmacist and Mrs. Smith initially regarding the label change.
- Mrs. Smith did not question the pharmacist about the potential incorrect strength.

Case 6.8

The mother of a 2-year-old child approached the dispensary and requested a bottle of Fer-In-Sol oral liquid. The pharmacy technician provided the 250-mL bottle of Fer-In-Sol Oral Solution Syrup, which contains 30 mg of ferrous sulfate per milliliter.

A few days later, the mother read the product label and immediately called the pharmacist to express her concern that the information on the product label did not match the information provided by the pediatrician. On investigation, it was determined that the pediatrician had intended that the child be given 1 mL of the Fe-In-Sol Oral Solution Drops, which contain 75 mg ferrous sulfate per milliliter or 2½ times the amount given.

Preventive Strategies for Nonprescription Medications

- Manufacturers should ensure that both the elemental iron and ferrous sulfate content are readily seen and understood by the public.
- Educate your patients about the relationship between elemental iron and ferrous sulfate. This also applies to ferrous gluconate, calcium carbonate, etc.
- Discuss label changes with your patients and the potential implications.
- Encourage your patients to ask questions, especially when something does not seem right.

IMMUNIZATION

Immunization prior to travel is an important public health priority. Immunization schedules often require personalized customization, depending on the countries to be visited, the type and duration of travel, as well as the amount of time available prior to departure. Patients, pharmacists, and physicians often overlook important details that may compromise the patient's ability to receive optimal immunization, as illustrated in Cases 6.9 and 6.10.

Case 6.9

A 66-year-old patient visited her physician in December for a regular checkup. During the visit, the physician asked the patient whether she was planning to travel during the winter months. The patient indicated that indeed she was planning a trip to Mexico with her daughter's family in March. The physician therefore wrote the following prescription and handed it to the patient.

Twinrix
Sig: As directed
Dispense: 3 doses

The patient took this prescription to her regular pharmacy for processing. On presenting the prescription to the pharmacy technician, the patient was informed that her insurance would not cover the cost of the vaccine. The patient indicated that since she did not need the vaccine immediately, she would keep the prescription and return later just prior to departing on her trip.

Two weeks before the trip, the patient returned with the prescription. The prescription was processed and dispensed correctly. During the counseling session, the pharmacist advised the patient of the primary course standard schedule of vaccination, consisting of the first dose now, the second dose 1 month later, and the third dose 6 months after the first dose.

The patient casually mentioned that she was looking forward to her trip to Mexico in 2 weeks' time. On hearing this, the pharmacist recognized that the time interval prior to departure would likely be insufficient to receive adequate protection against hepatitis A and B. The pharmacist therefore contacted the physician to discuss a change in the prescription to the rapid vaccination schedule, thereby increasing the level of protection. The rapid vaccination schedule consists of three injections given at 0, 7, and 21 days, with a fourth dose at 12 months after the first dose.

Case 6.10

Case 6.10 occurred in Canada, where the "Junior" formulation of Twinrix is available for patients 1 to 18 years of age. A physician wrote the following two prescriptions for a 45-year-old patient and his 13-year-old son:

Mr. Smith:

> *Twinrix*
> *Dispense: 3 doses*
> *Sig: As directed*

Jonathan Smith:

> *Twinrix*
> *Dispense: 3 doses*
> *Sig: As directed*

The standard vaccination schedule of Twinrix for an adult over 19 years of age is three doses at 0, 1, and 6 months.[6] However, the standard vaccination schedule for patients 1 to 18 years old is Twinrix *Junior* at 0, 1, and 6 months.

The pharmacist did not detect the prescribing error and therefore dispensed two Twinrix Adult doses as prescribed. The vaccines were taken directly to the doctor's office and were administered to both patients by the nurse.

Approximately a month later, the father returned to the pharmacy and requested the second Twinrix vaccine for both himself and his son. On this occasion, the dispensing pharmacist detected the prescribing, dispensing, and administration errors. The manufacturer of Twinrix was contacted to discuss the best course of action.

The pharmacist was advised to use the alternative vaccination schedule of Twinrix for patients 1 to 15 years old—that is, two doses of Twinrix *Adult* at 0 and 6 months.

A call was then made to the physician to discuss the issue and request the appropriate change to the prescription. The pharmacist also discussed the issue with the father and advised him that his son would require only one additional dose to be administered 6 months after the initial dose.

Possible Contributory Factors

- The prescriber and the initial dispensing pharmacist both assumed that Twinrix Adult would be appropriate for a 13-year-old.

- The nurse did not consider the appropriateness of the vaccine before administration.

Case 6.11

A 40-year-old patient took the following prescription to his local pharmacy for processing.

Twinrix   first dose now
Engerix-B   second dose at 1 month
Twinrix   third dose at 6 months

The patient asked that only the first vaccine (Twinrix) be dispensed. The remaining two vaccines (Engerix-B and Twinrix) were entered into the computer for future processing.

One month later, the patient returned and asked for his "second dose." On checking the patient's medication history it was assumed that the patient meant his second dose of Twinrix. The second Twinrix vaccine was therefore dispensed instead of the Engerix-B vaccine as prescribed.

Six months after his initial visit, the patient returned and asked for his "final dose." A check of the patient's medication profile revealed that only Engerix-B vaccine remained logged. The Engerix-B vaccine was therefore dispensed.

When the patient took the Engerix-B to the physician for administration, the error was detected. The patient was upset that the incorrect vaccine was dispensed and administered as the second dose.

Possible Contributory Factors

- The physician prescribed Twinrix and Engerix-B in a manner inconsistent with its approved labeling. According to the physician, the standard adult dosing schedule for hepatitis B vaccine (Engerix-B) is at 0-, 1-, and 6-month intervals. However, the hepatitis A vaccine (Havrix 1440) can be administered at 0 and 6 months. Therefore, in an effort to save the patient money, Engerix-B and not Twinrix was prescribed at the 1-month interval.

- The standard adult dosing schedule for Twinrix is at 0-, 1-, and 6-month intervals.[6] Therefore, on dispensing Twinrix at the 1-month interval, the pharmacist was adhering to the recommended dosing schedule and hence did not detect the error.

- The pharmacist that dispensed Engerix-B at the 6-month interval did not consider the dosing schedule of Engerix-B and Twinrix to confirm the appropriateness of the drug being dispensed.

- A copy of the original prescription was not readily available to the dispensing pharmacist when the second Twinrix vaccine was dispensed.

- The pharmacist who dispensed the original Twinrix vaccine did not make any notes in the patient profile regarding the unusual prescription.
- A lack of patient knowledge regarding his specific vaccination schedule.

Preventive Strategies for Immunization

- In dispensing vaccines, inquire whether the patient is planning a trip. If so, confirm the date of travel and determine whether there is sufficient time to complete the recommended dosing schedule.
- Patients should be advised to consult with their physician or travel clinic 2 to 3 months in advance of travel to allow for sufficient time for immunization schedules to be completed.
- Become familiar with the recommended dosage and vaccination schedule of the common vaccines.
- Before processing prescriptions, always obtain the patient's date of birth in order to confirm that all aspects of the prescription are appropriate.
- In dispensing vaccines, always consult an appropriate reference to confirm and adhere to the recommended vaccination schedule.
- Contact your software vendor to implement alerts that detect drug-age incompatibilities.
- In counseling patients, review the specific dosing schedule and the importance of adhering to this schedule. Suggest that they record the necessary dates on their calendar. Consider establishing a system whereby patients can be called to remind them of their next vaccine dose.
- If a prescription with an unusual dosage or dosing schedule is received, always contact the prescriber for clarification. Document the details of the discussion for future reference.
- Before dispensing "logged" prescriptions, always retrieve a copy of the original prescription. Technology exists whereby the original prescription can be scanned into the computer system and recalled on subsequent refills. Consider implementing this technology and discuss this with your software vendor.
- The following websites may be accessed for further helpful information:

  www.travelhealth.gc.ca
  http://wwwn.cdc.gov/travel/default.aspx
  http://www.who.int/ith/en/

METHADONE TREATMENT

One of the most widely used treatments for opioid-dependent individuals is pharmacological maintenance with methadone, an opiate agonist. Methadone is a synthetic opiate with good oral bioavailability and a long duration of action. Methadone blocks the euphoria produced by short-acting opioids, prevents withdrawal symptoms, and helps reduce drug cravings in opioid-dependent individuals.

Methadone maintenance typically involves the daily oral administration of methadone over an extended period of time as a long-acting substitute for heroin or other opioids.

Methadone is a safe medication when prescribed and consumed according to the guidelines in place, but it can be extremely dangerous when used inappropriately. Death has been reported with methadone doses as low as 50 mg in nontolerant individuals.[7]

Medication incidents involving methadone include:

- Administration of an incorrect dose
- Duplication of dosage
- Administration of a dose to the incorrect patient
- Methadone stock solution mistaken for water

Consider Cases 6.12 and 6.13, which illustrate incidents involving methadone.

Case 6.12

A 4½-year-old boy was prescribed amoxicillin suspension for cough and fever. Shortly after receiving the second dose of 5 mL, he became drowsy and less responsive. On admission to the emergency department, he was arousable only by deep pain, and pinpoint pupils were noted. A urine sample sent for a toxicology screen revealed the presence of methadone and its metabolite. Blood methadone concentrations were 0.23 and 0.14 mg/L 5 and 9 hours after the second dose of amoxicillin was given, respectively. The amoxicillin suspension was tested for methadone and was found to have a concentration of 2.4 g/L. The child gradually improved and was discharged on day 4 in good condition. The pharmacy in which the antibiotic had been dispensed was a dispensing center for a local methadone maintenance program, and methadone stock solution was accidentally mixed with the antibiotics instead of water.

Note: This case is reprinted with permission from Lalkin A, Kapur BM, Verjee ZH, Koren G. Contamination of antibiotics resulting in severe pediatric methadone poisoning. Ann Pharmacother. 1999 Mar;33(3):314–317.

Case 6.13

A busy community pharmacy dispenses methadone to approximately 40 patients on a daily basis. The doses are all prepared together ahead of time and stored in the refrigerator until the patient arrives to consume his or her dose in the presence of the pharmacist.

One Saturday, a 45-year-old patient arrived at the pharmacy for his observed dose of 70 mg methadone. The pharmacist opened the refrigerator and in error selected an incorrect bottle. The bottle selected contained a dose of 120 mg methadone for another patient. Without checking the label, the patient consumed the incorrect dose. After consuming the dose, the patient commented that the drink tasted stronger and more bitter than usual. On checking the label, the error was detected.

The pharmacist encouraged the patient to seek medical attention immediately; however, the patient refused. The patient said that he felt fine and did not want to spend hours waiting in the hospital. The pharmacist then attempted to contact the physician at his office but was unsuccessful. No emergency contact phone number was available for the physician. The pharmacist therefore counseled the patient to make sure that he was always in the presence of someone else who would be able to identify any signs of toxicity. The pharmacist also contacted the patient by phone on two occasions during the day to confirm that he was fine. Apart from excessive drowsiness, the patient did not appear to suffer any serious side effects.

The following day, a Sunday, the patient returned for his next dose. On this occasion, the pharmacist double-checked the label and confirmed that the patient was receiving the correct dose. The patient consumed the dose without incident.

Two days following the incident, the pharmacist contacted the physician to discuss the occurrence. Although the prescriber appreciated receiving the call, he was upset that he was not contacted immediately on his pager, which is always available for emergencies. He also expressed concern that the patient received his usual dose the next day following the incident. He explained that owing to the long half-life of methadone, the second dose could have been disastrous.

Preventive Strategies in Methadone Treatment

- If your pharmacy plans to dispense methadone, contact your licensing body to ensure that all the relative regulations and guidelines are known and adhered to.
- Ensure that all pharmacists and technicians on staff are appropriately trained in the dispensing and administration of methadone.
- Review and double-check all methadone prescriptions and dosages before they are administered. Whenever possible, have a second individual check the calculation and amount of methadone used in the preparation of the dose.
- Encourage physicians to write the methadone dose in words and numerals. The dose should be written in mg, not mL.
- When appropriate, use commercially available stock solution to reduce compounding errors.
- Prepare unique dosages at a different time and/or location to that used for the more common dosages.
- Contact other pharmacies experienced in the dispensing of methadone to identify potential pitfalls and strategies to avoid them.
- If you are compounding methadone solution from a powder, double-check and log the ingredient amounts independently. Place the finished product in a distinct bottle and clearly label it with the final concentration and date of preparation.
- Stock only one concentration of methadone if possible. If more than one concentration is required to manage patients, prominent warning labels should be used.

- In preparing daily doses, record and initial on the prescription hard copy the exact amount of stock solution used.
- Indicate on the prescription label of all dispensed unit doses the patient's name, the total dose, and the date of ingestion.
- Use a log to record the signature and proper identification of patients receiving witnessed and "carry" doses of methadone.
- Appropriate references should be up to date and accessible.
- Store all methadone solutions in a secure area separate from all other liquids.
- Consider storing methadone in separate, secure locations according to dosage (less than 50 mg), (50–100 mg), (more than 100 mg) out of patients' view.
- Serve one patient at a time in all circumstances.
- Implement appropriate methods of accurately identifying patients; for example, photo identification.
- Increase the font size of the patient's name and dosage on prescription labels.
- Maintain up-to-date contact information including emergency numbers for prescribing physicians.
- Implement a clear and succinct protocol for handling overdose. This should include but is not limited to the following:
  - Inform the patient that he or she has consumed an overdose.
  - Contact the physician immediately.
  - Strongly encourage the patient to go to the emergency room.
  - Explain why going to the ER is highly recommended (there is a high risk of death and the pharmacy is not equipped with a saturation monitor or a ventilator).
  - Ensure proper documentation of the incident.
  - Send all relevant information to the emergency room.

SUMMARY

Specialty practices can create unique challenges for the pharmacist in ensuring the safety of patients. In this chapter, effective preventive strategies are discussed for specialty practices, including pediatrics, compounding, nonprescription medications, immunization, and methadone. In addition to the application of the many recommendations discussed, innovative technology can also be used to maximize efficiency and enhance patient safety. These technological advances are discussed in the following chapter.

Reflective Questions

1. For pediatric patients, discuss ways to double-check dosages based on the child's age and weight.
2. Review your current practice with respect to potassium chloride. Identify ways that your procedures can be enhanced to improve patient safety.
3. Identify nonprescription medications with problematic names, packaging, or labeling. Discuss ways to educate patients about these products so as to improve safety.

4. What steps can be taken to ensure that patients adhere to their recommended immunization schedule?
5. Review the methods currently used to manage dosing errors involving methadone. What improvements could be implemented in your methadone practice to enhance patient safety?

REFERENCES

1. Abraham C. Dosage errors imperil children: study. Globe and Mail, April 11, 2002.
2. Levine SR, Cohen MR, Blanchard NR, et al. Guidelines for preventing medication errors in pediatrics. *J Pediatr Pharmacol Ther.* 2001;6:426–442.
3. Repchinsky C, ed. Compendium of Pharmaceuticals and Specialties. Ottawa: Canadian Pharmacists Association; 2007:499.
4. Jew RK. Extemporaneous Formulations. Philadelphia: Children's Hospital of Philadelphia; 2003.
5. Extemporaneous Oral Liquid Dosage Preparations. Toronto: Canadian Society of Hospital Pharmacists; 1988:3–6.
6. Repchinsky C, ed. Compendium of Pharmaceuticals and Specialties. Ottawa: Canadian Pharmacists Association; 2006:2289.
7. Harding-Pink D. Methadone: One person's maintenance dose is another person's poison. *Lancet.* 1993;341:665–666.

Chapter 7

Technology Solutions to Promote Safe Medication Practices

Objectives

After completing this chapter, the reader will be able to:

- Recognize the types of automation technologies that can assist in minimizing dispensing errors and improving patient safety
- Identify the advantages and disadvantages of each potential technology
- Understand how changes to the workflow process can help reduce potential errors
- Recognize the environmental and operational factors that can lead to inefficiencies and dispensing errors
- Implement a plan of action to prevent dispensing errors

As discussed in the previous chapters, medication incidents can occur at multiple points during the process of creating and interpreting the order and then preparing, dispensing, and administering the medication. Some of these medication incidents come from "role overload" and job stress caused by workloads that the individuals involved may feel are more than they can manage. In one survey, more than 60% of respondent pharmacists reported that equipment and/or technology increased the level of their productivity and the quality of care provided to patients, and about half reported that it increased their job satisfaction.[1]

The implementation of technological solutions has great potential for minimizing medication incidents by reducing the possibility of human error in the prescribing, dispensing, and administration processes and giving clinicians more time to spend on cognitive services such as increased patient counseling. Potential technological solutions include the following:

- **Computerized physician order entry**
- Computerized decision support
- Computerized prescription transmission systems
- Telephone management systems
- Bar coding for medication order entry
- Dispensing and administration
- Workflow software

- Automated dispensing machines
- Unit-dose systems/compliance packaging
- Point-of-care medication administration

Technology can be used to reduce medication incidents at each step in the prescribing, dispensing, and administration process. Physician prescribing can be enhanced by the use of computerized order entry, **decision support,** and electronic transmission of prescriptions; also, telephone management systems may be used for refills. At the dispensing stage, workflow software ensures that each and every prescription is handled identically (and adheres to desired standards). Bar coding of product, unit-dose systems, and automated dispensing equipment can virtually eliminate the chance of dispensing the wrong product or the wrong strength of the right product. At the drug administration stage, bar coding can again help to ensure the "five rights" of medication administration safety: right patient, right medication, right route, right time, and right dose.[2]

This chapter reviews some of the technologies that have the largest potential to have a positive impact on patient safety.

COMPUTERIZED PHYSICIAN ORDER ENTRY (CPOE)

One of the most error-prone areas of prescription filling involves deciphering the physician's handwriting. Written orders can also be incomplete and ambiguous. Given this danger, in 2000 the Institute for Safe Medication Practices (ISMP) called for the abandonment of handwritten scripts by 2003—a goal that is obviously still far from achievement.[3]

CPOE systems are electronic prescribing systems that are primarily used in hospitals. They permit physicians to enter orders directly into a computer rather than writing them on paper. Electronic communication of prescriptions allows for a more accurate conveyance of the prescriber's intent.

There are different levels of systems. The most complex and effective can also offer real-time decision-making support to the physician by offering background information on prescribing guidelines, such as evidence-based guidelines (either national or hospital-specific) and instant access to drug information. This information is crucial, given the increasing complexity of drug therapies available and of individual patients' drug regimens.

The software programs are structured so that no field is left empty: dosage, frequency, and all other pertinent information must be filled in. If the clinician does not enter all of the required data, the system will suggest the best possible choice of frequency or dosage for the clinician to approve. CPOE, along with decision-support software, can reduce the likelihood of incidents during the prescription ordering process in a number of ways. A CPOE system may include the following[4]:

- Provides information regarding drug of choice and appropriate alternatives
- Provides feedback regarding medication appropriateness and formulary availability
- Provides information about potential drug duplication

- Checks for patient-specific information such as allergies, age, and weight
- Screens for drug–drug or drug–disease interactions
- Recommends appropriate dosages
- Provides high/low dose warnings
- Reviews patient medication history

CPOE Systems' Impact on Patient Safety

CPOE systems produce legible prescription orders that include all required information and avoid the use of possibly confusing abbreviations.[5] These systems can also save time, because pharmacy staff no longer needs to transcribe the prescription into the pharmacy's system and do not have to waste time calling the physician to clarify indecipherable or incomplete orders.

CPOE systems have been shown to be remarkably effective in reducing the rate of serious medication incidents. A study conducted by Bates et al. at a large tertiary care hospital demonstrated that CPOE reduced serious medication errors by 55%, from 10.7 events per 1,000 patient-days to 4.86 events per 1,000 patient-days.[6] In another study, Bates et al. concluded that CPOE resulted in a significant decrease in the frequency of medication incidents (excluding missed-dose errors) most likely to harm patients.[7] In a study of pediatric patients, researchers conducted a prospective trial of 514 pediatric patients admitted to a 20-bed pediatric critical care unit in a tertiary care children's hospital before and after the implementation of CPOE. They reviewed all medication orders during the study period (a total of 13,828 orders). Before the implementation of CPOE, 2.2 potential adverse drug events (ADEs) and 30.1 medication prescribing errors (MPEs) occurred per 100 orders. After CPOE, potential ADEs were reduced to 1.3, and MPEs were reduced to 0.2 per 100 orders. The overall error reduction was 95.9%.[8]

In addition to reducing the risk of incidents, CPOE can also influence the selection of the right drug and right dose. An analysis was conducted of all adult inpatient orders at a U.S. medical center where all orders were entered through a CPOE system. When orders are entered, the system displays drug use guidelines and suggests appropriate doses and frequencies. With the computerized guidelines, the use of the recommended drug (nizatidine) increased from 15.6% of all histamine-blocker orders to 81.3%. The proportion of doses that exceeded the recommended maximum dose decreased from 2.1% before CPOE to 0.6% thereafter.[9]

The Leapfrog Group have made the claim that CPOE can reduce errors by 50%, and these and other studies clearly show that the Leapfrog Group's claim is conservative.[10] Indeed, when decision-support features are added to a CPOE system, medication errors can be reduced up to 81%.[11]

Limitations of CPOE Systems

Despite its many benefits, CPOE has not been widely implemented. In a recent study of the approximately 6,000 hospitals in the United States, it was estimated that only 9.6% have fully implemented CPOE.[12]

At the time of writing, a large number of these systems were not interfaced with the pharmacy management system; thus the information must be re-entered into the pharmacy system. However it is hoped that this is temporary and will become rarer with time. In a hospital setting that phases in CPOE, pharmacy may come late in the game; but even in those cases where the pharmacist would be forced to re-enter the prescription, at least it would not be a scribble. Legibility would not be an issue.

Barriers and Challenges to CPOE

Barriers and challenges to the implementation of CPOE include the following:

- Financial commitment
- Physician and staff acceptance
- Training
- Interorganizational communication
- Introduction of "new errors" due to new technologies

The financial commitment to install and maintain a CPOE system and to train staff is significant. Bates estimated the cost for developing and implementing CPOE at Brigham and Women's Hospital, an academic tertiary-care hospital with approximately 700 beds, to be $1.9 million (USD), with maintenance costs of $500,000 per year.[13]

Physician acceptance is also a key element to successful implementation. If the decision-support system places too many demands on the physicians' time, clinical judgment, or decision making, they may reject its use. Obtaining buy-in from physicians usually requires their involvement during the entire process, from analysis through implementation. The pharmacy department and hospital management also need good leadership and communication skills to ensure that all staff understand the benefits of this type of system.

Physicians may delegate the order entry to other staff, such as nurses. In these cases, other staff still have to key in the information manually, negating CPOE's benefits and potentially opening the door to additional errors because of nonphysician entry. One study compared the rate of order-entry misses or near misses made by physicians and nonphysicians at two sites. The rate of errors committed by nonphysician computerized order entry was much higher than that associated with physician order entry. The researchers suggested that non-physicians might not be able to recognize problems such as potential interactions and inappropriate routes of administration.[14]

Operators may see review messages or alerts regarding drug use as excessive and confusing and so may frequently override them. As well, operators who are nonphysicians may not be capable of correctly interpreting the alert messages provided by the system.

Administrators must plan for sufficient training time and obtain buy-in from all staff to ensure that they see the system as a benefit and not just another burden in their already full schedules. In addition, and applicable to all technologies covered in this chapter, the facility's information services department must be capable of handling the demands of planning, implementing, and maintaining the new technologies.

There is a lack of standards for representation of most types of key clinical data. As a result, applications do not communicate well even within organizations, and the costs of interfaces are high.[15] In an effort to address this issue, the ISMP has developed "Draft Guidelines for Safe Electronic Communication of Medication Orders."[16] Discussion of this issue is ongoing among industry and caregivers.

New types of errors will inevitably be created, including "point and click" errors, where prescribers choose the wrong drug from on-screen menus, or errors created by remote CPOE, where the prescription is entered without the patient's chart in hand. In one reported case, this led to a medical resident prescribing a Norcuron (vecuronium) infusion for the wrong patient.[17] In one study, 22 types of medication error risks were associated with the system.[18] The authors grouped these as (1) information errors generated by fragmentation of data and failure to integrate the hospital's several computer and information systems and (2) human–machine interface flaws reflecting machine rules that do not correspond to work organization or usual behaviors.

Too many alerts, irrelevant pop-ups, and slow computer response times are often encountered, making it harder for staff to embrace the new technology.

A software-only solution that combines CPOE with formulary support does not address the two critical phases of dispensing and administration, which together account for nearly 50% of medication errors.[19]

E-PRESCRIBING

In the community setting, physicians may use **e-prescribing** (or electronic prescribing) software. The theory is the same as with CPOE: rather than writing a potentially illegible script by hand, the physician enters the order electronically into a computer, which is then sent to a pharmacy for dispensing.

E-prescribing is available on a number of levels. At the most basic, it would involve a stand-alone writer, with no access to patients' medication histories or supporting data. At the most complex, it could involve a system that includes all of the patient's medical information, formulary information, medication management systems, connectivity between other providers such as pharmacies and insurers, and integration of the device's data with the patient's complete health file in the physician's office.[20]

When "writing" a prescription, the prescriber uses an electronic pad with fields for treatment indications. Once the electronic prescription order is complete, the prescriber sends a copy to a secure server and, in some cases, prints out a hard copy for the patient. The pharmacist then downloads this prescription, using an access code located in the patient's file or on the patient's copy of the prescription. The prescription then becomes part of the pharmacy system. Any subsequent stop and/or change orders are transmitted to the pharmacy that dispensed the prescription. Depending on the system in use, new and change orders may be transmitted immediately or in batches. If they are transmitted in batches, patients may arrive at the pharmacy before their prescriptions are available to the pharmacy system.

E-prescribing programs can also provide:

- A list of the current prescriptions and medications purchased within the previous 12 months
- A list of all drugs prescribed by the physician from his or her handheld device
- A color-coded classification of drugs prescribed by the treating physician and those prescribed by other physicians (confidentiality rules may prevent this from happening unless the patient has consented to this sharing of information)
- A refill compliance calculator
- Dates of emergency room visits and hospital admissions
- Cost of drugs dispensed

Advantages of E-Prescribing

Some of the advantages of these programs for pharmacists include:

- Decreased time spent on prescription clarification and less chance for medication incidents
- Less time spent on clerical tasks, freeing up the pharmacist's time to focus on patient care
- The provision of automatic electronic prescription updates and medication stop/change orders, which increases the timeliness of care
- Greatly improved communication and cooperation between pharmacists and physicians

The Medical Offices of the XXIst Century (MOXXI) research project being conducted at McGill University in Montreal is testing the benefit of implementing an electronic prescription, drug, and disease management system.[21] It integrates basic e-prescribing programs with downloadable patient profiles as well as sophisticated decision tools that are founded on evidence-based, peer-reviewed clinical guidelines.

Each physician in the project receives a personal digital assistant (PDA) with MOXXI software, including electronic health records for each participating patient as well as an alert system that detects interactions between drugs, inappropriate drug dosages, treatment duplications, and contraindications. (For more information about MOXXI, go to www.moxxi.mcgill.ca/moxxihome.html.)

Barriers and Challenges to E-Prescribing

While e-prescribing greatly reduces the likelihood of a pharmacist misinterpreting a physician's drug order, these devices are only as good as the information programmed into them. For example, the most perfect reproduction of a physician's order is useless if the physician created the wrong order in the first place (e.g., chose a suboptimal drug, dose) because of a "point-and-click" error or because the relevant guidelines were not available or were not used. Also, if a patient is seeing a number of different physicians, each of whom has prescribed different medications, information about all of these drugs may need to be input into the device before it can check for drug–drug interactions.

It is clear that the successful implementation of CPOE systems and e-prescribing can reduce medication incidents at the prescribing stage; however, the drug administration phase remains vulnerable. Hence, incident reduction efforts must look beyond these systems in order to achieve maximum patient safety.

BAR CODE TECHNOLOGY

A bar code is a machine-readable symbol, usually composed of bars and spaces, which can be found on most consumer products. As part of drug labels, the bar code could contain a variety of different types of information, including the National Drug Code (NDC), package size, dosage form, lot number and expiry date. The bar code would enable health professionals to use computerized databases to verify that the correct drug is being dispensed and/or administered. This is especially beneficial in avoiding incidents where two products have similar packaging or NDCs (as seen in Chapter 4).

Bar codes, placed on staff identification badges or on wristbands worn by staff, can be used to identify team members involved in the various stages of the dispensing process, such as computer entry, filling, checking, and patient counseling.

In addition to their time-saving benefits (scanning a bar code vs. reading and re-entering alphanumeric data), bar codes reduce errors inherent in manual data entry and, at the dispensing and administration stages, bar coding offers the potential to reduce medication incidents.[22]

Although bar code technology has been available and widely used for many years in the grocery and retail sector to manage inventory and document transactions, it has not been widely adopted in the health care sector to reduce medication incidents associated with drug products.[23,24] According to a 2000 ISMP Medication Safety Self-Assessment, 43% of hospitals had discussed the possibility of bar coded drug administration, but only 2.5% used this technology in some areas of the hospital and less than 1% had fully implemented it throughout the organization.[25]

In order to fully reap the benefit of bar coding, it is essential that staff avoid taking shortcuts with the system. For example, in picking up two packages of the same product, staff must remember to scan each package individually rather than scanning the same bar code twice. The use of workflow software designed to recognize and disallow double scans of the same medication would avoid reliance on staff remembering and following management directives.

Advantages of Bar Coding

The U.S. Food and Drug Administration (FDA) estimates that the bar code rule, once implemented, will result in a 50% increase in the interception of medication incidents at the dispensing and administration stages. This would result in 413,000 fewer adverse events over the next 20 years in the United States.[26]

Bedside bar coding, where both the patient's bracelet and chart bar codes are scanned at the time of dispensing, is a simple means of ensuring the right drug is dispensed to the right patient.[27]

Hospitals that have implemented bar code technology have seen significant decreases in medication incidence rates.[28] The Veterans' Affairs Medical Center of North Chicago reported an 86% drop in medication incidents in the first year after implementing a bar code system.[29]

Bar codes, placed on staff identification badges or on wristbands worn by staff, allow tracking which staff members were responsible for each dispensing function for each prescription, thus allowing functions such as the overriding of allergy alerts to be restricted to pharmacists only.

Bar codes can also be used in community pharmacies to confirm that the prescription has been dispensed with the correct drug.[30]

Challenges and Limitations of Bar Code Technology

Currently, there are a number of obstacles to the full implementation of bar code technology. These include the following:

- Not all drug packaging contains the manufacturer's bar code. Items repackaged in unit doses, injectable vials, and IV admixtures often lack bar codes. Pharmacies must therefore create and add their own bar codes to some drug products. However, the cost of producing bar codes can be prohibitive for many pharmacies.
- Health care providers may be resistant to the implementation of new technologies and changes to workflow processes. Successful implementation requires the buy-in of staff with appropriate education and training.
- There may be high costs associated with the implementation of bar code technology.
- There is a lack of uniform electronic standards.

However, these and other challenges can be overcome with the coordinated efforts of all stakeholders, including the pharmacy profession, health care institutions, governments, and manufacturers.

RADIO FREQUENCY IDENTIFICATION

Radio frequency identification (RFID) tags are similar to bar codes but can be used in instances where bar codes are inappropriate (for example, because of a small package size). These tags can be as small as a fingernail and as thin as a millimeter. They consist of a computer chip that can be read when passed through an electronic field.

Tags on patient bracelets can be used to identify hospital inpatients or hospital staff, just as bar codes are. The tags could include information such as the patient's allergies, current medications, and recent lab results. All of this information could be updated or revised whenever needed. In future, it is even possible that each individual pill could have its own tag embedded inside, ensuring even more exact and safe medication administration.[31]

The focus for RFID at present is to deter theft and counterfeiting as well as to improve product availability, inventory management, and the product recall process. These requirements make RFID use throughout the dispensing process more affordable and will increase and further enhance patient safety.[32]

AUTOMATED DISPENSING

There are a wide variety of automated dispensing systems available for both community and hospital pharmacies; these may be implemented to enhance patient safety and improve productivity and efficiency of the pharmacy.

Types of Automated Dispensing Systems

There are two types of automated dispensing systems: centralized and decentralized, with the latter more prevalent in hospital pharmacy.

Centralized Dispensing Systems

Centralized dispensing systems such as robotics use bar code technology to automate all aspects of the dispensing process, including the storage, dispensing, returning, restocking, and crediting of bar coded unit-dose medications. Robotic systems can select and count the required drug, choose a vial, label the vial, place the drug into the vial, and deliver the labeled vial to the pharmacist for checking.

On-screen imaging of the drug being dispensed can assist with visual verification. Many of these systems are also capable of providing a scanned image of the original written or electronic prescription. This image is displayed to the dispensing pharmacist each time the prescription is being refilled. This can prevent one or more repetitions of an original dispensing error.[33]

The robotic system is useful mainly for reducing incidents related to drug dispensing and administration.[34] By reducing time-consuming dispensing, checking, and distribution tasks, these systems can free up the pharmacist's time to focus on patient-care activities.

Decentralized Systems

Decentralized systems such as unit-based cabinets in hospitals can be used to automate the storage, dispensing, and tracking of floor stock, narcotics and scheduled medications as well as PRN medications in the patient care area. Figure 7.1 shows an example of a medication dispensing cabinet—AcuDose Rx—available from McKesson Provider Technologies. One study conducted in a 600-bed hospital identified a reduction in the number of medication errors with an automated dispensing unit (10.4%) compared with the control

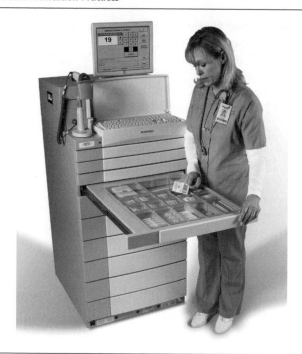

FIGURE 7.1 AcuDose R$_x$. (Courtesy of McKesson Provider Technologies.)

(16.9%).[35] In both study phases, most of the errors were wrong-time errors. Both the decrease in the error rate and the decrease in the departure from scheduled administration times were statistically significant.

Centralized and decentralized technologies can be used individually or in combination. As well, they can be linked to other technologies such as CPOE and point-of-care administration systems (described below) to create a closed loop of patient care. Automated dispensing systems in hospitals, if connected with the physician and pharmacist electronic files, may decrease medication incidents by ensuring the medication is administered on the floor exactly as the doctor prescribed it.[36]

Benefits of Automated Dispensing

Automated dispensing machines are available for both community and hospital pharmacies and may vary in their complexity depending on the practice site. However, they both provide similar benefits:

- Problems with look-alike/sound-alike drugs can be avoided.
- The mechanical aspect of the job is removed, thus freeing up time for more counseling and other patient care services.
- Less time is wasted, as automated dispensing removes the chance of the wrong drug being picked up. This avoids the need to correct that error at a later stage in the dispensing process. Even where no injury is involved, errors often create extra work, and the costs involved may be substantial.[37]

OTHER TECHNOLOGIES THAT CAN REDUCE MEDICATION ERROR RATES

There are a variety of other technologies that can reduce medication error rates, including interactive voice response (IVR), queuing management systems, wireless communications, workflow software, vertical carousels, tablet counters, automated dispensers, robotics, strip packaging machines, automated water dispensers, automated will-call systems, near infrared (NIR), central fill, electronic health records, and talking vials. Each of these is discussed briefly here.

Interactive Voice Response

Interactive voice response (IVR) and its derivatives, including automatic validation in host and automatic doctor communications, reduce errors by allowing patients to enter their refill prescriptions via the Internet or their phone's keypad, bypassing the verbal communication to a pharmacy staff member (and the subsequent manual notation and data entry). Automatic validation within the pharmacy management system can be instantaneous, ensuring that the prescription is valid and has refills available. If communication with the patient's doctor is required, many systems have the ability to handle those needs via fax or e-mail without involving pharmacy staff. IVR systems also have the ability to help with patient compliance through automated follow-up calls and refill reminders. In hospital settings, a telephone follow-up 2 days after hospital discharge reportedly allowed pharmacists to identify and resolve drug-related problems for 19% of patients.[38,39] IVR reduces interruptions and distractions to the dispensary staff, further reducing the risk of medication incidents.

Queuing Management Systems

Queuing management systems allow facilities to manage patient flow, helping to reduce the peaks and valleys of the workday (and workload). Queuing systems also allow pharmacies to decide whether to fill prescriptions in the traditional format or in a 'bank teller' mode. In bank-teller mode, patients wait for an available pharmacy staff member (usually at a service window) and then have all their prescriptions filled while they wait at the window (where they also receive counseling). By managing patient flow and allowing for flexible approaches to pharmacy practice, queuing systems reduce stress and related errors. Figure 7.2 illustrates a queuing system screen in a busy waiting area.

Wireless Communications

Cordless headsets for phones allow pharmacy staff members to speak on the phone while keeping their hands free to take notes and retrieve or enter data. Some wireless devices allow pharmacy staff to automatically find associates within the pharmacy or on the hospital campus or else automatically route the request to voice mail.[40]

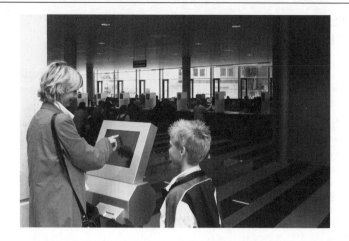

FIGURE 7.2 Queuing Management. (Courtesy of Q-Matic Corporation.)

Workflow Software

At its best, workflow software allows pharmacy staff to work in an environment where the technology ensures that each prescription is filled following the same steps, with the same checks and balances, as all others. It would include the ability to map and remap[5] products within the pharmacy—separating look-alike/sound-alike drugs and reducing the risk of incidents as described in Chapter 4.[41] "Mapping" refers to the software's ability to store and print/display the location of all items within the pharmacy. This reduces the time it takes to locate and retrieve product and leads to the ability to remap the pharmacy. Remapping involves relocating products within the pharmacy both to save time and to reduce potential errors. Placing often used products closer to filling and seldom used products farther away can provide significant timesaving benefits. It also allows for the separation of multiple strengths of the same medication (and of sound-alike products) to reduce potential errors.

Workflow software is accessed completely by bar code scans and enables bar code verification of product selection; it may provide "red screen" warnings and images of both the original hard copy and the product being dispensed. Workflow software should also automate order grouping, allowing technicians to fill prescriptions as they arrive without concern for keeping patients' prescriptions together. Letting the system regroup patients' prescriptions and schedule prescriptions based on urgency allows technicians to work at a faster pace and reduces clutter on the filling counter (which could lead to dispensing errors). Finally, the software should be able to locate an individual prescription at any stage of the process. Example screens from a workflow software system—Innovation's Symphony—are shown in Figure 7.3.

Vertical Carousels

Vertical carousels allow for medication storage that optimizes space efficiency and provides error reductions by utilizing bar code scanning and pick-to-light

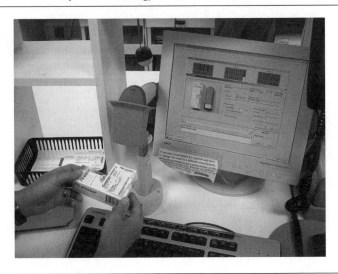

FIGURE 7.3 Symphony Workflow Screenshots. (Courtesy of Innovation.)

technologies. A bar code scan sets the shelves revolving until the shelf containing the product is available. The product itself is identified by a light under its location. An example of a vertical carousel, McKesson Provider Technologies' MedCarousel, is shown in Figure 7.4. One study documented a 96% reduction in dispensing errors, from an average of 42 errors per week to 1.8 through the use of vertical carousels.[42]

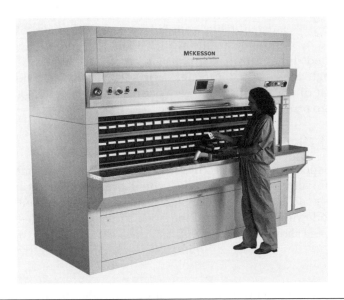

FIGURE 7.4 MedCarousel. (Courtesy of McKesson Provider Technologies.)

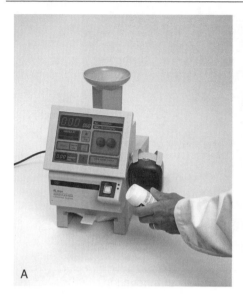
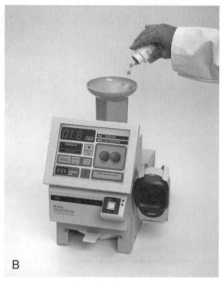

A   B

FIGURE 7.5 KL16. (Courtesy of Kirby Lester, LLC.)

Tablet Counters

"Universal" or 'countertop" tablet counters (where the stock is poured into the patient's vial in a weigh-type machine or stock is poured through a machine into a scoop) now use bar code scanning to verify the stock bottle retrieved matches the product (and strength) requested by matching it to a bar code on the prescription label set. These counters also eliminate errors that occur when a manual count is interrupted. An example, Kirby Lester's KL16, is shown in Figure 7.5.

"Cassette" or "canister" tablet counters (where each high-volume product is stored in its own unique canister which is then placed on a counting unit) can be activated directly from the pharmacy's management system, allowing validation that the correct canister was placed on the counting unit. Replenishment of the canisters also uses bar code verification against the stock bottle to ensure error-free dispensing.

Automated Dispensers

Automated dispensers are also activated directly from the pharmacy computer and, unlike universal or cassette styles, count product directly from product-specific storage cells. As with canister systems, replenishment of the cells requires bar code verification against the stock bottle. An example—Innovation's SmartCabinet—is shown in Figure 7.6.

Robotics

Robotics choose a vial, print the label, apply the label to the vial, count the required medication and place it in the vial. Some then cap the vial before

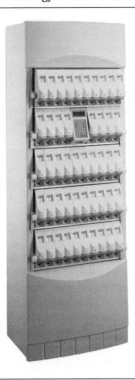

FIGURE 7.6 SmartCabinet. (Courtesy of Innovation.)

presenting to the pharmacist for checking. As with automated dispensers (above), bar code verification is crucial during replenishment. ScriptPro's SP200 is shown in Figure 7.7.

Strip Packaging Machines

Strip packaging machines—formerly used only for long-term care facilities—are now being used for patients of all ages who prefer their medications in compliance pack strips. (Strip packagers are covered below in the "Unit Dose Systems" section.)

Automated Water Dispensers

Automated water dispensers eliminate errors of the incorrect volume of water added to the drug powder, thereby resulting in an inaccurate concentration of drug being dispensed as well as errors where the wrong liquid is used to reconstitute.[43] Systems are available that use bottled pharmacy grade water as well as systems that use their own reverse osmosis (R/O) filtration systems. Most are equipped with bar code scanners that read the stock-bottle bar code and display the product name and strength on their screen as well as the recommended volume of water. If accepted by the pharmacy staff member, the system dispenses an initial portion of the total quantity, requests (on screen) that the product be

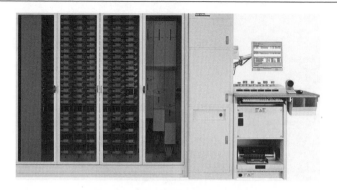

FIGURE 7.7 ScriptPro SP200. (Courtesy of ScriptPro.)

mixed, and then dispenses the remaining volume. If the R/O system is not used, bar code verification on replenishment should be required.[44] Figure 7.8 shows an example, Serinor's $R_x$econ.

Automated Will-Call Systems

Will-call can be improved, and errors reduced, with partial or completely automated will-call systems. Partially automating involves using pick-to-light systems, while full automation is provided by systems that store and retrieve patient's orders via bar code scans. Most automated will-call systems are still located within the pharmacy and are under pharmacy control at all times; however, new systems are being developed that allow the patient to enter a personal identification number and electronic signature to obtain a prescription after the pharmacy has closed.[45] What all formats have in common is the reduction or elimination of the right product(s) going to the wrong patient(s).

Near Infrared (NIR)

Near infrared (NIR) is an emerging technology worth noting. In the testing stages at the time of this writing, NIR spectroscopy is able to identify the unique "fingerprint" of the medication being dispensed. The initial focus for NIR was to identify counterfeit drugs; however the technology is also being tested as a device to provide an additional check for pharmacists or, in some mail order facilities, as a potential replacement for pharmacist verification.[46,47]

Central Fill

While not a single "product" in the sense of the above technologies, central fill offers an alternative form of dispensing that has the potential to provide significant error reductions. Central fill or central refill centers use economies of scale to allow for extreme levels of automation. Most use all of the aforementioned technologies (and much more) to fill prescriptions for multiple sites (either under single or multiple ownerships).[48]

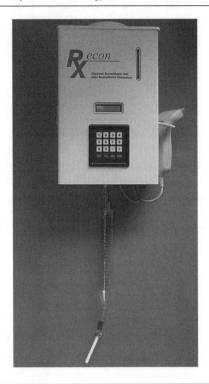

FIGURE 7.8 R$_x$econ. (Courtesy of Serinor.)

Through their use of high technology, these facilities allow pharmacists to check (right product and strength only) 1,000 prescriptions per hour while maintaining a total facility error rate (wrong product to patient) of less than 0.0006%.[49]

Electronic Health Records

The Electronic Health Record (EHR) is an electronic record containing all patient health information, including:

- Patient demographics
- Past medical history, including immunizations
- Laboratory data
- Radiology reports
- Progress notes
- Vital signs
- Medications

The EHR automates and streamlines intra and interdepartment workflow and can be interfaced with evidence-based decision support, quality management, and outcomes reporting.

Winner of a 2005 Award for Medication-Use Safety, Evanston (Illinois) Northwestern Healthcare reported that since implementing the electronic record, they have eliminated 100% of all transcription-related errors and have seen a 70% decrease in delayed administration of medications to patients, a 20% decrease in omitted medication administration, and a 50% reduction in time from order to administration of first-dose antibiotics.[50]

Talking Vials

The ScripTalk Audible Prescription system was selected in 2005 as the sole audible prescription-reading device that the U.S. Department of Veterans Affairs (VA) facilities can now purchase for patients. According to the Veterans Health Administration (VHA) directive on audible prescription-reading devices, a pharmacist must test each label to ensure that the audio matches the visual, although that may change as newer versions of these devices are released. One such advance captures data on its way to a traditional printer, converts the data stream to speech, and records it to the medication vial.[51]

LIMITATIONS OF TECHNOLOGY IN MEDICATION ERROR REDUCTION

While technology has great potential to improve the quality of care for patients, it may also introduce new risks into the medication provision process.

- There is concern with some automated systems that nurses on the hospital unit will override the system to obtain the drug more quickly (e.g., because of time constraints or a lack of understanding of the system).
- Pharmacy staff might be tempted to slacken their vigilance and depend too much on technology to catch errors. Care must be taken to stay alert for potential medication incidents, and monitor systems to uncover any new risks.[52]
- It is important to have strategies in place to deal with prescription orders during "down times" (e.g., during power failures, or when the system is down because of routine maintenance, system backups, or upgrades).
- The time required for staff education and training often exceeds what was originally expected.[53]
- The addition of technology affects facilities design. If an experienced design/automation consultant is not used, the technology's value may be reduced.

AUTOMATION CASE STUDY

The flowcharts shown in Figure 7.9 illustrate the prescription filling process with and without the technologies discussed in this chapter. The unshaded boxes indicate areas where human decision making may lead to errors, while the shaded boxes indicate steps where technology now provides checks and balances—mostly via bar code scans.

    Using a combination of workflow software and multiple levels of counting equipment, a high-volume U.S. Department of Defense outpatient pharmacy reduced MEDMARX (USP national database for medication errors) reported errors by 59%.[54] In addition to the significant improvements in patient

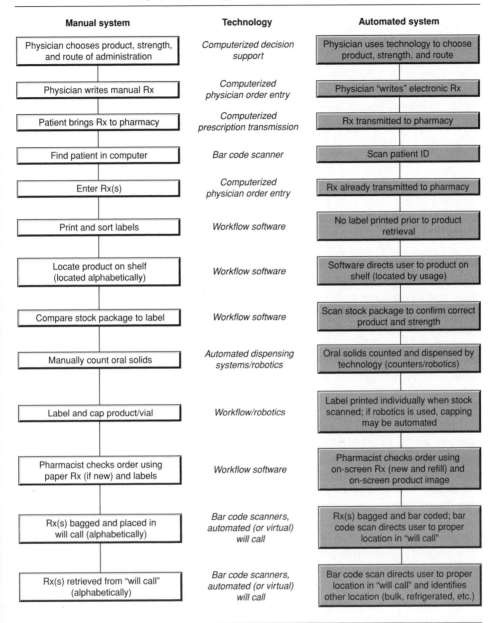

Manual system	Technology	Automated system
Physician chooses product, strength, and route of administration	*Computerized decision support*	Physician uses technology to choose product, strength, and route
Physician writes manual Rx	*Computerized physician order entry*	Physician "writes" electronic Rx
Patient brings Rx to pharmacy	*Computerized prescription transmission*	Rx transmitted to pharmacy
Find patient in computer	*Bar code scanner*	Scan patient ID
Enter Rx(s)	*Computerized physician order entry*	Rx already transmitted to pharmacy
Print and sort labels	*Workflow software*	No label printed prior to product retrieval
Locate product on shelf (located alphabetically)	*Workflow software*	Software directs user to product on shelf (located by usage)
Compare stock package to label	*Workflow software*	Scan stock package to confirm correct product and strength
Manually count oral solids	*Automated dispensing systems/robotics*	Oral solids counted and dispensed by technology (counters/robotics)
Label and cap product/vial	*Workflow/robotics*	Label printed individually when stock scanned; if robotics is used, capping may be automated
Pharmacist checks order using paper Rx (if new) and labels	*Workflow software*	Pharmacist checks order using on-screen Rx (new and refill) and on-screen product image
Rx(s) bagged and placed in will call (alphabetically)	*Bar code scanners, automated (or virtual) will call*	Rx(s) bagged and bar coded; bar code scan directs user to proper location in "will call"
Rx(s) retrieved from "will call" (alphabetically)	*Bar code scanners, automated (or virtual) will call*	Bar code scan directs user to proper location in "will call" and identifies other location (bulk, refrigerated, etc.)

FIGURE 7.9 Comparison of prescription filling process with and without technology. (Courtesy of Efficient Pharmacy Solutions.)

safety, they reported substantial reductions in prescription processing time, specifically:

- A 13% reduction in average patient processing time
- Substantial reductions in prescription fill times (ranging from 40%–62% savings depending on which automation was in use)

UNIT-DOSE SYSTEMS

At the drug administration stage, the unit-dose system of drug distribution has great potential to reduce the risk of medication incidents. In these systems, single doses of medications are packaged in a ready-to-administer form for a specific patient. Before being dispensed, the medication order is reviewed by a pharmacist to ensure it is appropriate. However, if an error does occur in the preparation and labeling of the dose, the effect of the error is limited, since unit-dose medications are generally supplied for a 24-hour period only. A study conducted at Toronto's Hospital for Sick Children showed a reduction in medication incident rate from 10.3% to 2.9% when the traditional drug distribution system was replaced with a unit-dose system.[55]

In contrast, access to bulk medication by nonpharmacists on the hospital floor or the dispensary after hours can lead to medication incidents. In one reported case, hydralazine 10 mg IV q6h prn was prescribed for a patient. In error, a nurse removed a hydroxyzine 25-mg vial from a dispensing cabinet, drew up 10 mg, and gave the dose IV push. Hydroxyzine should be given IM only, not IV, owing to the risk of tissue necrosis if the drug is accidentally injected subcutaneously or intra-arterially. In this case the patient suffered no adverse outcome.[56]

At the community pharmacy level, medications are often dispensed in blister packs, Dosettes, or multidose compliance packs to enhance patient compliance. Elderly patients are especially at risk of noncompliance due to their often complex medication regimens. The blister packaging, Dosette, or multidose compliance pack must be clearly labeled to identify its contents. The packaging and labeling of these compliance aids must also be carefully checked by the pharmacist to prevent dispensing incidents. Since the compliance aids are usually not child-resistant, special care must be taken to ensure that children cannot access the medication.

Newer to community pharmacy is strip packaging, usually using automated high-speed packagers. Figure 7.10 shows McKesson Provider Technologies' PacMed system. These systems reduce cost (versus blister packaging or Dosettes) and allow greater flexibility in the way medications are provided to the patient, thus improving compliance and allowing nurses or other caregivers to spend more time with patients. Strips may be unit-dose, multidose, or a combination of the two (with certain products packaged separately). Pouches can be supplied sorted by administration time or by product and, in long-term care environments, can be sorted by ward and administration time. Empty pouches can be used as reminders (e.g., time for eyedrops, inhaler, or a refrigerated product).

Although unit-of-use packaging is not widely employed in the United States, it is commonplace in other countries—bringing with it important safety and usage benefits.[57] Strip packaging is growing in popularity among all age groups and ambulatory levels, with high growth expected from patients who travel frequently as well as in the provision of manufacturers' product samples.[58] One community pharmacy, having installed a high-speed packager to handle its long-term care market, transferred 15% of its ambulatory patients to strip packaging in the first 3 months.

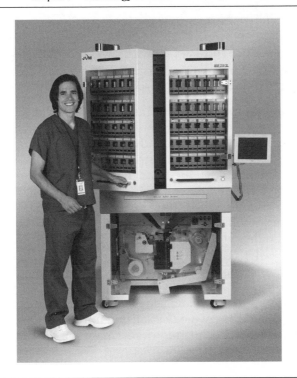

FIGURE 7.10 PacMed. (Courtesy of McKesson Provider Technologies.)

POINT-OF-CARE MEDICATION ADMINISTRATION SYSTEMS

Point-of-care medication administration systems utilize bar code technology to ensure that the right patient receives the right dose of the right drug at the right time via the right route (the five rights) can be seen as the last line of defense against incidents at the patient's bedside. They may involve a variety of device options, including handheld and full-screen laptop versions.

When the nurse is administering a drug, he or she first selects the patient's name from a computer device or scans the bar code attached to the patient's identification wristband. The nurse also scans the personal identification bar code on his or her name tag as well as the medication bar code. The software checks the patient's medication profile for potential administration errors. If no errors are identified, the medication is administered and a real-time medication administration record is automatically created. However, if a potential error is identified, the nurse receives an alert message.

Advantages of Point-of-Care Systems

Point-of-care medication administration systems reduce the potential for medication incidents and the associated patient harm, costs, and liabilities by:

- Prohibiting the option to bypass the "five rights" of verification
- Providing critical data monitoring

- Providing warnings and alerts to prevent potential medication incidents before they occur
- Requiring a hospital staff member to witness the administration of critical drugs, as determined by the hospital
- Providing multiple alert messages based on discrepancies

In an observational study conducted at the University of Wisconsin Hospitals and Clinics, a point-of-care medication administration system was used and a comparison was made of errors before and after implementation of the technology. The result showed medication administration errors were reduced by approximately 87%.[59] Errors identified included the incorrect drug, dose, dosage form, time of administration, and missed doses. Another study at the Department of Veterans Affairs reported a similar (86.2%) reduction in reported errors. Despite these positive outcomes, researchers also found a substantial number of instances where users overrode valid warnings and administered doses that differed from the written order (although 70% of the events the system identified as possible errors were without merit, supporting the users' decisions to override the warnings).[60]

This technology provides many benefits, including reduced administration errors, improved scheduling of medication and improved efficiencies, increased drug-monitoring efficiency, and improved communication among the health care team.

THE IMPACT OF FACILITIES DESIGN

One of the factors that influence human error is our psychological well-being. Stress and fatigue result in enormous losses of productive time and an elevated risk of error.[61] The recognition and alleviation of stress and fatigue can help to reduce error rates as well as help to retain and attract new employees and patients.

One way to reduce patient pressure and pharmacist stress is to provide a comfortable waiting area for patients. Many pharmacies are adding children's play areas to the waiting area to help parents keep young children occupied. Another waiting area idea to consider, especially as our patients continue to age, is to have multiple small waiting areas throughout the pharmacy.

The design within the pharmacy dispensing area is also crucially important to relieving stress. Poor arrangement of workflow disrupts pharmacy staff, resulting in distractions that can lead to errors. Some of the signs of poor workflow include employees bumping into each other or having to excuse themselves to pass; insufficient counter space; and overflowing shelves. These all result from design flaws that will cause decreased productivity, inefficient movements, and an increased risk of process errors.[62]

Other design or environmental factors that can have an influence on error rates, as discussed in Chapter 5, include:

- Inadequate lighting[63]
- Ambient noise levels[64]

- Poor ventilation[64]
- Temperature and humidity[64]
- Color (of the walls, counters, cabinets, and fixtures)[65]
- Music[66,67]

As technology is introduced into the workplace, proper placement of the technologies must be considered in relation to the above environmental factors and design changes may need to be implemented. Failure to take these steps will reduce the efficiency of the technologies.[68]

SUMMARY

Technology has the power to help the health care team reduce and prevent medication incidents. In an ideal world, all possible technologies would be implemented. However, with scarce resources, difficult choices must be made among the available technologies. Health care professionals must evaluate the beneficial impact on medication incidents as new technologies are implemented and must also continue to remain vigilant for the potential for incidents.

Reflective Questions

1. Review the technologies presented in this chapter and categorize them based on whether they are potential short- or long-term goals for your practice. Discuss with coworkers and management to ensure the list is complete and properly prioritized.
2. Using these two lists, identify which of the technologies (not yet in use) are most likely to help you reach your goals.
3. Discuss the feasibility of implementing those new technologies and identify short- and long-term strategies for their implementation.
4. Via the Internet, access some of the referenced articles on design and environmental factors and note where your practice area(s) may be deficient.
5. Using Figure 7.9 as a template, prepare a flowchart of your prescription filling process and note areas where human decision making adds potential for errors.

REFERENCES

1. Anon. Heavy workloads still an issue, but pharmacists' satisfaction improves. *Drug Store News.* 2006;14:18
2. Anon. Incorporating safe medication principles into daily practice. ASHP research and educational foundation. 2004. Available at: http://symposia.ashp.org/medsafety/Exercise_book_For_Nurses.pdf. Accessed January 2007.
3. Anon. A call to action: eliminate handwritten prescriptions within 3 years! Electronic prescribing can reduce medication errors. 2000. Available at: www.ismp.org/newsletters/acutecare/articles/whitepaper.asp?ptr=y. Accessed January 2007.

4. Briceland L. Reducing medication errors through advances in automation. American Society of Health-System Pharmacists 35th midyear clinical meeting. Available at: www.medscape.com/viewarticle/418385. Accessed June 28, 2004.

5. Davis NM, Cohen MR. Computer-generated prescription orders. *Am Pharm.* 1995; NS35(9):10.

6. Bates DW, Leape LL, Cullen DJ, et al. Effect of computerized physician order entry and a team intervention on prevention of serious medication errors. *JAMA.* 1998; 280(15):1311–1316.

7. Bates DW, Teich JM, Lee J, et al. The impact of computerized physician order entry on medication error prevention. *J Am Med Inform Assoc.* 1999;6(4):313–321.

8. Potts AL, Barr FE, Gregory DF, et al. Computerized physician order entry and medication errors in a pediatric critical care unit. *Pediatrics.* 2004;113(1 Pt 1):59–63.

9. Teich JM, Merchia PR, Schmiz JL, et al. Effectiveness of computerized physician order entry on prescribing practices. *Arch Int Med.* 2000;160:2741–2747.

10. Anon. Effect of CPOE on medication errors. *Am J Health-Syst Pharm.* 2006;63:409.

11. Zhan C, Hicks RW, Blanchette CM, et al. Potential benefits and problems with computerized prescriber order entry: analysis of a voluntary medication error-reporting database. *Am J Health-Syst Pharm.* 2006;63:353–357.

12. Ash JS, Gorman PN, Seshadri V, et al. Computerized physician order entry in U.S. hospitals: results of a 2002 survey. *J Am Med Inform Assoc.* 2004;11(2):95–99.

13. Bates DW, Leape LL, Cullen DJ, et al. Effect of computerized physician order entry and a team intervention on prevention of serious medication errors. *JAMA.* 1998;280: 1311–1316.

14. George D, Austin-Bishop N. Error rates for computerized order entry by physicians versus non physicians. *Am J Health-Syst Pharm.* 2003;60(1):2250–2252.

15. Bates DW, Gawande AA. Improving safety with information technology. *N Engl J Med.* 2003;25(348):2526–2534.

16. Anon. It's time for standards to improve safety with electronic communication of medication orders. Institute for Safe Medication Practices. Newsletter. *Acute Care.* 2003; (Feb 20). Available at: www.ismp.org/Newsletters/Acutecare/Articles/20030220.asp. Accessed November 2006.

17. Institute for Safe Medication Practices. Remote CPOE error—a situation that's more than remotely possible. Available at: www.ismp.org/Newsletters/acutecare/articles/20070531.asp. Accessed October 30, 2007.

18. Koppel R, Metlay, J, Cohen A, et al. Role of computerized physician order entry systems in facilitating medication errors. *JAMA.* 2005;293(10):1197–1203.

19. Posey LM. Point-of-care technology to reduce hospital medication errors. *Pharm Today.* 2006;(Jan):7.

20. Electronic Prescribing Initiative. Electronic prescribing: toward maximum value and rapid adoption. Washington, DC: eHealth Initiative; 2004;(April 14):12. Available at: www.ehealthinitiative.org/initiatives/erx/document.aspx?Category=249&Document=269. Accessed February 28, 2008.

21. Tamblyn R. Towards an integrated delivery system for optimal drug management—challenges and solutions for the new millennium. Moxxi PMA Phase III Report. Presented at Canadian Association of Chain Drug Store (CACDS) conference; 2002.

22. Caverly WM. Bar coding: save time and reduce errors. *Efficient Pharm.* 1999;2(3):2–4.

23. Brussel E. Barcodes and the dispensary. *Efficient Pharm.* 1998;1(2):4.

24. Cina J, Fanikos J, Mitton P, et al. Medication errors in a pharmacy-based bar-code-repackaging center. *Am J Health-Syst Pharm.* 2006;63:165–168.

25. Anon. The supermarkets do it—so why can't we raise the "bar" in health care? *ISMP Med Safety Alert.* July 25, 2001. Available at: www.ismp.org/MSAarticles/supermarket.html. Accessed October 2004.

26. FDA proposes drug bar code regulation. Available at: www.fda.gov/oc/initiatives/barcode-sadr/fs-barcode.html. Accessed June 27, 2004.

27. Cohen MR. Medication errors. *Am Pharm Assoc*. 1999;11–18.

28. Young D. FDA proposes bar codes on drugs. *Am Soc Health-Syst Pharm*. Bethesda, MD, 13 March 2003. Available online: www.ashp.org/news/ShowArticle.cfm?id=3345. Accessed June 27, 2004.

29. Ault A. FDA told bar codes on drugs would cut errors. Available at: www.medscape.com/viewarticle/439347. Accessed June 27, 2004.

30. Stewart I. Focus on error prevention. Bar coding technology. *CPJ*. 2003;136(4):16.

31. Chaiken B. Playing tag to enhance patient safety. Patient Safety & Quality Healthcare. 2004. July/Sept. Available at: www.psqh.com/julysep04/tech.html. Accessed October 2, 2004.

32. Vecchione A RFID: Ready for prime time in 2006? *Drug Topics*. 2006;149:59.

33. Fitzgerald WL, Wilson DB. Medication errors: lessons in law. *Drug Topics*. 1998;142:84–91.

34. Murray MD. Automated medication dispensing devices. In: Markowitz AJ, ed. Making Health Care Safer: A Critical Analysis of Patient Safety Practices, Evidence Report/Technology Assessment Number 43, July 20, 2001. Rockville, MD. Available at: www.ahrq.gov/clinic/ptsafety/chap11.htm. Accessed October 8, 2004.

35. Borel J, Rascati K. Effect of an automated, nursing unit-based drug-dispensing device on medication errors. *Am J Health-Syst Pharm*. 1995;52:1875–1879.

36. Oren E, Shaffer ER, Guglielmo BJ. Impact of emerging technologies on medication errors and adverse drug events. *Am J Health-Syst Pharm*. 2003;60:1447–1458.

37. Young D. IOM: US drug errors harm 15 million annually. *ASHP News*. Available at: www.ashp.org/s_ashp/sec_news_article.asp?CID=167&DID=2024&id=16096. Accessed Januray 2007.

38. Ling C. What was said. *Solutions in Drug Plan Management*. May 12, 2005.

39. Timm Wagner L, Kenreigh C. Computerized physician order entry: fallible, not foolproof. Medscape Web site. November 17, 2005. Available at: www.Medscape.com/viewarticle/516367. Accessed November 2006.

40. Gebhart F. Pharmacy thrives in all-digital hospital. *Drug Topics*. 2005;149:13.

41. Caverly WM. Improving efficiencies and reducing medication errors. Part 2. *Efficient Pharm*. 2000;3(3):1–4.

42. Ragan R, Bond J, Major K, et al. Improved control of Medication use with an integrated bar-code-packaging and distribution system. *Am J Health–Syst Pharm*. 2005;62:1075–1080.

43. Stewart I. Reconstituted pediatric antibiotics: Vague directions can lead to problems. *CPJ*. 2005;138(8):66.

44. Caverly WM. Technology watch: liquid dispensers. *Efficient Pharm*. 2000;3(1):2.

45. Alexander A. Pharmacy kiosks gaining momentum. *Drug Store News*. 2005;27:37.

46. Kirsche ML. Drug "fingerprints" may halt counterfeits, say Md Researchers. *Drug Store News*. 2004;26:27–32.

47. Polli JE, Hoag SW. Near-infrared technology detects counterfeit drugs. *US Pharm*. 2004;29(2):104.

48. Tammaro J. Central fill: is it in your future? *Efficient Pharmacy*. 2001;4(3):2.

49. U.S. Department of Veteran Affairs. VA CMOP update 2007. Available at: www.amsus.org/sm/presentations/Feb07-A.ppt#256,1,Department of Veterans Affairs. Accessed October 30, 2007.

50. Perry L. Three health systems recognized for drug safety. Drug Topics Health-System Edition. 2005;149:HSE4.

51. Thompson C. Audible medication vials slowly gain momentum. *Am J Health-Syst Pharm*. 2005;62:116–119.

52. Coleman B. Hospital pharmacy staff attitudes towards automated dispensing before and after implementation. *Hosp Pharm.* 2004;11:248–251.
53. Wellman GS, Hammond Rl, Talmage R. Computerized controlled-substance surveillance: application involving automated storage and distribution cabinets. *Am J Health-Syst Pharm.* 2001;58:1830–1835.
54. Caverly WM. Department of Defense Outpatient Pharmacy Impact of Automation study. 2003 unpublished study done by McKesson APS for the U.S. Navy.
55. O'Brodovich M, Rappaport P. A study of pre and post unit dose conversion in a pediatric hospital. *Can J Hosp Pharm.* 1991;50:5–15.
56. Anon. Let us know if "tall man" letters have been effective. *ISMP Safety Alert.* 2003; 8(19):3.
57. Apsden P, Wolcott J, Bootman JL, et al, eds. Preventing Medication Errors: Quality Chasm Series. Committee on Identifying and Preventing Medication Errors. Board on Health Care Services. Institute of Medicine of the National Academies. Washington, DC: The National Academies Press; 2006. Available at: http://www.iom.edu/CMS/3809/22526/35939.aspx. Accessed January 2007.
58. Anon. U.S. pharmaceutical packaging demand to reach $6.8 billion in 2008. *Packaging Digest.* Available at: www.packagingdigest.com/bytes/pharm.php. Accessed January 2007.
59. Puckett F. Medication-management component of a point-of-care information system. *Am J Health-Syst Pharm.* 1995;52(12):1305–1309.
60. Sakowski J, Leonard T, Colburn S, et al. Using a bar-coded medication administration system to prevent medication errors in a community hospital network. *Am J Health-Syst Pharm.* 2005;62:2619–2624.
61. Caverly WM. Stressed and tired? *Pharm Post.* 2001;9(1):21.
62. Caverly WM. Improving efficiencies and reducing medication errors, part 4. *Efficient Pharm.* 2001;4(1):1–3.
63. Caverly WM. See pharmacy design in the right light. *Pharm Post.* 2000;8(1):22.
64. Caverly WM. Create a hospitable indoor climate. *Pharm Post.* 2000;8(8):17.
65. Caverly WM. Room for colour in pharmacy. *Pharm Post.* 2000;8(6):18.
66. Caverly WM. Whistle while you work. *Pharm Post.* 2001;9(5):37.
67. Caverly WM. Music to our ears, dollars in our pocket. *Pharm Post.* 2001;9(10):31.
68. Caverly WM. Walk this way. *Can Pharm J.* 2002;135(8):46.

Chapter 8

Dealing with Medication Incidents in Pharmacy

Objectives

After completing this chapter, the reader will be able to:

- Develop a plan for dealing with a medication incident
- Explain a protocol for handling a medication incident
- Describe and complete an incident reporting form
- Define and describe root cause analysis
- Demonstrate how to handle a medication incident using an appropriate process and communication techniques

The previous chapters in this book are directed at preventing medication incidents; however, it must be accepted that because of human error and all the contributors to error that have been discussed thus far, medication incidents will likely continue to occur, although one must hope to a minimal degree. James Reason has said that even highly reliable organizations expect to make errors.[1] The workforce must therefore be trained to recognize and recover from them.[1] All levels of the organization must be equipped to deal with errors and know how to convert setbacks into improved safety of the system.[1]

Having accepted that incidents will occur, a pharmacy or pharmacy organization should have a plan of action to deal with incidents. This involves many issues, including patient relations, legal implications, regulatory requirements, human resources, and public relations. The appropriate handling of the incident with the patient and later with pharmacy personnel is critical to prevent negative outcomes such as punishment, legal repercussions, and personal distress. It is helpful to have a protocol that pharmacy staff members are prepared to follow while using appropriate communication techniques. This can help ease the process and reduce negative outcomes. It will ensure that the incident is handled appropriately, the patient is sensitively treated, and similar incidents are prevented from recurring.

Medication incident reporting is a critical element of handling an incident that was ignored until recent years, resulting in recurrence of often fatal incidents. Incidents should be reported at several levels, including personal, pharmacy department, organizational, and national to ensure the most benefit.

Finally, the incident should be investigated through a **root cause analysis** to identify both root and immediate causes and develop strategies to prevent future incidents from occurring.

149

PLAN OF ACTION FOR HANDLING A MEDICATION INCIDENT

The way that an incident is dealt with is critical to the outcome and to the value of any lessons for the prevention of recurrences. In many cases, it is the mishandling of an incident that leads to a complaint to a pharmacy regulatory body or to legal action. A plan of action for handling a medication incident should be made and shared with all staff so that it is clear how to proceed prior to incidents occurring. A plan of action for handling a medication incident should include the considerations summarized in Table 8.1.[2–6]

An Appropriate Person Should Oversee Handling

An appropriate person should have responsibility for overseeing the handling of a medication incident and ensure that appropriate communication and follow-up of the incident occurs. In a community pharmacy, the pharmacy owner or manager should have this responsibility. Initially, the pharmacist—not a technician—should communicate with the patient concerning medication incidents. In the case of a serious incident resulting in patient injury, the owner or manager should become involved to offer further apologies and possibly calm the situation. In a larger organization, there may be a designated person in authority who is trained to deal with incidents. There may also be a committee which sees that an incident is properly handled and investigated. Even so, in the case of a serious incident resulting in patient harm, the individuals involved should communicate directly with the patient to offer an apology for any inconvenience or distress.

When an incident comes to light, it may be difficult for the pharmacist to remember on the spot all the details of how a medication incident occurred. The pharmacist should be given a reasonable amount of time to collect his or her thoughts and review what happened before communication or further

---

TABLE 8.1
Plan for Handling a Medication Incident

- The appropriate person should deal with the situation
- Follow a suggested protocol
- Be open and honest
- Inform the appropriate people
- Communicate fully with the patient
- Complete reports and investigation
- If necessary, deal with the media
- Communicate with staff
- Insure that recommended actions are taken to prevent recurrence
- Deal with insurance issues

investigation proceeds. The pharmacist should write down his or her recollection of the incident as soon as possible. This should help to avoid self-contradiction later and will show credibility. However, the incident should be dealt with and discussed as soon as possible so that environmental and psychosocial contributors can be recognized and documented.

Follow a Suggested Protocol

It is helpful to follow a set protocol for handling medication incidents and communicating with patients. It can help to reduce the stress of a situation when all the pharmacy staff members know exactly how to proceed in case of an incident, and it also reduces the chances that the situation will be mishandled. Some pharmacy employers have recommended protocols, as do some pharmacy regulatory bodies and insurers. A suggested protocol is discussed in a later section of this chapter.

Be Open and Honest

Most importantly, to start with, the pharmacist should be open and honest, with both the patient and any investigating bodies about the incident that has occurred.[5] In fact, it has been common for patients involved in incident investigations to make comments such as, "If the pharmacist had been up front instead of trying to cover up his mistakes, I would never have lodged a complaint."[5]

It should be recognized that investigations by regulatory bodies are not intended to determine guilt or innocence but rather to protect the public by investigating complaints in an unbiased manner.[5]

The principle of disclosure has become a cornerstone of handling medical errors. Previously, health care providers were warned to avoid making apologies to patients because it might lead to problems if they were sued.[7] Today it is considered compulsory for an institution to have a disclosure policy that includes acknowledgment of medical errors. A disclosure program called the "three Rs," for "Recognize, Respond, and Resolve," was instituted for physicians in Colorado in 2000 and resulted in a 50% decrease in malpractice claims.[7] A similar program, "Sorry Works!", was instituted in Illinois.[7]

Inform the Appropriate People

When an incident occurs, both internal and external people need to be notified. Internally this would include management of the pharmacy (in the pharmacy and head office of a chain pharmacy) and other staff. Externally, the physician should be informed when a serious incident has occurred or if there may be any effect on the patient, since it may also affect the physician's interpretation of patient symptoms; for example, missed doses resulting in poor symptom control. There should also be communication with the patient, reporting of the incident to reporting programs, notification to the insurer (if harm has resulted) and to a regulatory body if action will be taken in this regard.

The plan should make clear who provides the notification, internally and externally, what the time line is for notification (e.g., within 24 hours), and what information should be given. There may be several stages to this communication, including an initial verbal report of an incident, followed up with completion of an incident reporting form, root cause analysis, and outcomes and recommendations from the investigation. At all times, privacy and confidentiality should be considered regarding the patient and pharmacy staff members involved.

Communicate with the Patient

As part of open and honest disclosure, the patient should be informed. If possible, this should be directly with the patient rather than through an intermediary such as a family member, who may not be fully aware of the patient's circumstances and may be less forgiving than the patient. All discussions with the patient should take place in a private area so that other patients do not overhear what has happened and become concerned themselves. Similarly, any discussion about the incident within the pharmacy or institution should be kept private and confidential.

Even if it is unclear where the cause of the incident originated or if any harm resulted, a full apology for any inconvenience or upset that has been caused should be made by the pharmacist and the pharmacy or institution. This is not an admission of guilt or blame but rather an apology for any effect on the patient.

The pharmacist should ensure the patient's welfare. He or she should ask whether the patient ingested the wrong medication and calmly provide appropriate information about the potential outcome. If necessary, the patient should be advised to seek further advice or treatment from his or her physician or emergency services. A follow-up contact should be made with the patient to inquire about any further outcome.

The patient should be assured that a full investigation will be made to determine what went wrong and that everything possible will be done to see that it will not happen again. Once the root cause analysis is complete, the patient should be informed in an appropriate manner of the identified causes of the incident and the actions that will be taken to prevent recurrences.

Further details of communication with the patient are discussed in a later section of this chapter.

Complete Reports and Investigate

The pharmacy should investigate and resolve the incident as soon as possible. An incident report should be completed and root cause analysis conducted (to be discussed in later sections of this chapter). This should be done in a transparent manner so that the patient is aware that it is being conducted. If this does not appear to be happening, the patient may feel compelled to report to a body of higher authority (e.g., the head office of a pharmacy chain or a regulatory body).

Dealing with the Media

In the case of a serious medication incident, there may be news media inquiries. If left up to the media to investigate, they may not arrive at all the facts or possibly misconstrue them. As noted above, disclosure is now considered necessary, but it can be done in a positive and controlled manner if it is well planned and anticipated. There should be a plan for who should answer the questions and how; for example, whether the hospital or pharmacy chain public relations department or a designated spokesperson should be the respondent. The media should be told that an investigation is being conducted and a report summarizing the results of that investigation will be communicated when it is complete. Confidentiality should be maintained for the people directly involved in the incident, but accurate information should be disclosed.

Communicate with Staff

As a learning exercise, all pharmacy staff members should be made aware of the occurrence of a medication incident. They should be involved in the root cause analysis and informed of any outcomes relating to policy or procedures to prevent recurrences. Confidentiality of staff directly involved in the incident should be maintained to encourage reporting of incidents. Further issues relating to staff involved in a medication incident are discussed later in this chapter.

Make Sure That Recommendations to Prevent Recurrence are Implemented

When the investigation into a medication incident is complete, there should be a summary of recommendations. This may include policy implementation, new design of procedures or facilities, and other actions. There should be a plan in place to ensure that these occur in a timely manner, including how and when they will be implemented. In this way lessons from the incident will not be lost and recurrence will, one hopes, be prevented.

Deal with Insurance Issues

Pharmacists should be certain that they are properly insured for individual (not just pharmacy) liability and know what their insurance clause requires. It may require the pharmacist to notify the insurance company immediately in case of a problem, and the insurance company may suggest a procedure to follow. The pharmacist's employer may also have an insurance policy or procedure to be followed.

PROTOCOL FOR HANDLING A MEDICATION INCIDENT

Depending on the pharmacy setting, medication incidents may be handled slightly differently, but in either community or institutional settings it is important that a preplanned protocol be understood and followed by all involved.

A suggested protocol for handling a medication incident in community pharmacy is shown in Figure 8.1.

How a medication discrepancy is dealt with initially depends on whether it is reported by a patient or it is identified by pharmacy staff members. If it is identified in the pharmacy, the incident should be verified; then the patient

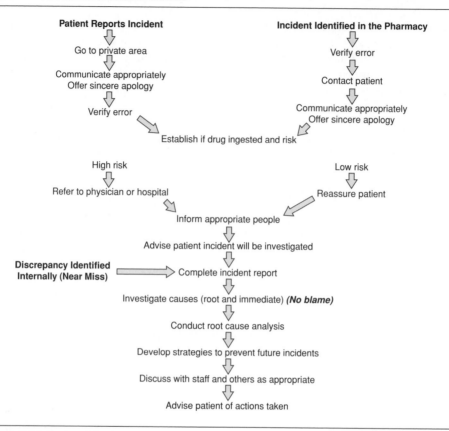

FIGURE 8.1 Protocol for handling a medication incident.

must be contacted and appropriate communication and an apology should be made to inform the patient of the incident (as discussed above).

If the patient identifies the discrepancy, the pharmacist should escort the patient to a private area of pharmacy to discuss the issue. Appropriate communication and a sincere apology should be made for any concern or inconvenience. As discussed earlier, this is not an admission that an error has been made or an admission of guilt at this point.

An inquiry should then be conducted to verify the incident by, for example, comparing the contents of the medication container with the drug name on the label; comparing the original hard-copy prescription with the label for drug name, dosage form, strength, quantity, and directions; and checking the patient's history to determine if a different strength or dosage had previously been used. The pharmacist should determine whether any changes were made intentionally. If a discrepancy is not evident following this inquiry (e.g., if a change in medication noted by the patient was actually intended) the patient should be thanked for inquiring and assured that it was not a bother to verify the right medication. This encourages patients to be vigilant and knowledgeable about their medications, as they are important partners in preventing medication incidents, as discussed in Chapter 3. If, however, a discrepancy is verified, the patient should be informed of this in an open and honest way.

It is critical at this point to determine whether the drug was ingested, and if so whether there is any risk to the patient. If so, the patient should be referred to the hospital or his or her physician and appropriate measures taken. If there is no risk to the patient, he or she should be reassured of this, but the incident should not be trivialized.

Whether the incident is discovered by the patient or a pharmacy staff member, the appropriate people should be informed, as noted earlier. Communicating with the patient is the most important step. To start, a sincere apology should be made—regardless of whether the medication was dispensed by the pharmacist handling the incident or by another pharmacist or technician. If another pharmacist dispensed the medication, the patient should be assured that all staff will be informed. As soon as possible, the other pharmacist involved should also be informed. If the incident is serious, it may be advisable for the pharmacist involved to also speak with the patient and apologize. If necessary, the physician should be contacted at this point and informed of the incident (communication with the physician is discussed later in this chapter).

If a discrepancy occurs whereby the error was identified internally prior to reaching the patient (i.e., a near miss), then the protocol should be followed from this point on so that it is still reported and a root cause analysis is conducted to prevent the discrepancy from occurring again and potentially reaching a patient next time.

Next, an incident report should be completed. It is important to assure the patient that the incident will be investigated. Completing the incident report is the start of the root cause analysis from which strategies can be developed to prevent future similar incidents. The final report, along with recommendations, should be communicated to all staff and any other parties in the system who may have contributed to the cause of the incident, (e.g., the manufacturer regarding confusion of sound-alike product names; the physician regarding ambiguous directions).

Finally, the patient should be informed of the actions that will be taken to prevent further incidents.

INCIDENT REPORTING

It has been said that the establishment of a reporting culture is crucial to effective risk management.[1] Incident reporting is critical to improving patient safety. The main goal of such a reporting program should be to learn as much as possible about the immediate and systemic causes of medication errors and, through that, to understand how to prevent harm to patients.[8] Reporting programs have the following goals[9,10]:

- To identify common types and causes of medication incidents
- To determine trends and track data
- To raise awareness and guard against future incidents
- To gather information for the root cause analysis

- To identify causes of errors in systems and processes
- To identify ways to prevent recurrent events

It has been suggested that incident reporting should be mandatory and as such serve to hold providers accountable for performance and patient safety; however, this is in conflict with the concept of a "no-blame" system.[9] The Institute for Safe Medication Practices (ISMP) recommends that reporting be voluntary, in order to encourage reporting, since the main values of reporting, as stated above, depend on having all incidents reported. Mandatory reporting programs tend not to be successful because reporting is inconsistent and therefore unreliable.

The ISMP also cautions about the use of incident reports to benchmark or compare individuals, departments, or institutions because of differences in the culture of organizations, patient populations, definitions of a medication error, and differences in the types of reporting and detection systems used.[8] However, accumulating anonymous data about medication incidents can identify significant problems, such as product issues (sound-alike, look-alike, and packaging issues), system design, or human resources issues. This allows organizations to lobby for changes that are in the purview of other organizations, such as regulatory bodies, government, or pharmaceutical manufacturers. It also allows for wide distribution of warnings and alerts about common problems.

Reporting needs to be completed by front-line practitioners at the time of occurrence so that important information about what happened and why can be reliably reported, including environmental and psychosocial conditions.[9]

Implementing Incident Reporting

All staff members need to know how to report a medication incident or discrepancy (near miss), including what forms are used, who should complete the report, what should be reported, and when. What is considered reportable should be very clearly stated so that no one can make excuses for not reporting. The report should be completed by the individual who discovers the error. It should be completed as soon as possible, so that all details can be remembered and root cause analysis can be started without delay.

All efforts should be made to encourage and persuade pharmacy staff members to submit reports. There are, however, significant disincentives to reporting, including fear of discipline, loss of license or job, legal repercussions, embarrassment, and the extra time and work involved. In order to ensure that reporting occurs, the reporting itself must be a confidential and nonpunitive process. The ISMP has identified best practices to promote error reporting, including the following[10]:

Ensure Confidentiality

Names of staff involved must be on the form, along with the pharmacist handling the incident, the time and location of the incident, and the patient's identity in order for proper analysis to be completed. However it is crucial that those handling the report keep this information strictly confidential; once the report has been investigated, names are removed.[10] It must be clear to all pharmacy staff that the information will be kept confidential.

Demonstrate Trustworthiness

Individuals involved in medication incidents must feel that they can trust the people who will be receiving the report, whether it is a manager, a committee, or a formal reporting agency. This can be established only by clear statement by the reporting program managers that the purpose of reporting is to improve patient safety and not to punish or judge; by evidence that reports are used for the purposes stated and changes are made as a result; by evidence that reporters are not treated unfairly or in any way punished; and that confidentiality is maintained as discussed above.

Take Clear and Quick Action

When pharmacy staff see that reports they have made are used to remove potential risks and improve safety, they are likely to feel that the time and effort they have taken was worthwhile. Feedback should be provided as soon as possible about the root cause analysis and recommendations as well as implementation plans for those recommendations.

Recognize Efforts of Reporters

Pharmacy staff members who submit reports should be acknowledged by the program managers and thanked for taking the time and effort to do so. Ideally, there would be incentives for reporting, such as extra pay for the time involved.

Make It Easy

The reporting process must be simple and clear to all. If possible, it should allow a variety of reporting mechanisms, including electronic, oral, and written. It should ask specific questions rather than broad, general questions, allowing the reporter to describe what happened in his or her own words. It should also list various options of causes, such as communication problems, labeling, drug storage, environmental, etc., to assist the reporter in recording all possible causes. It should be easy to submit a report and require minimal time, so that it will be done as soon as possible after the event, aiding memory of details that may be crucial to root cause analysis.

Ensure a Culture of Safety

As discussed in Chapter 3, it must be clear to all pharmacy staff that patient safety is everyone's ultimate goal and responsibility and that the organization is committed to this. This should be discussed with all new staff and proper training provided about patient safety and the importance of being part of prevention, including reporting incidents or near misses. This is discussed further in Chapter 9.

Deal with Staff Fairly

When a medication incident is reported, no punitive actions should be taken, unless negligence, harmful behavior, or malign intent is apparent (e.g., drug or alcohol abuse by the employee/employees involved; failure to follow policies, procedures, guidelines, or regulations).[11] It should be made clear that the purpose of following up is not to assign blame but rather to make it a learning process for everyone, even those who were not involved in the incident. Value should be placed on the reporting and learning aspect, so that those who report such incidents are congratulated for their efforts rather than made to feel ashamed[10] (see also later discussion of staff issues).

Safeguard against Litigation

An important factor that may deter some people from making a report is fear of litigation. There is concern that any records of a medication incident could be used as evidence against a pharmacy staff member in a court case.[3,4] It has been the case that disclosure has exposed organizations and individual practitioners to penalties in terms of financial, professional, and public scrutiny. On the other hand, having a complete report of the circumstances, outcomes, and actions taken following an incident may be critical during any kind of legal challenge. In some jurisdictions, regulatory or legislative allowances have been made to make medical error reporting free of risk of litigation in order to encourage incident reporting and thus ultimately improve patient safety.

In order to safeguard against records being inappropriately used in this regard, for example for use as evidence in a law suit against an individual, the following recommendations have been made[3,4]:

- Keep the incident report separate: details of the incident should not be attached to the medical file. The medical effect should be recorded in the patient's medical record, including only the facts and a description of the patient's response over at least 24 to 48 hours following the incident.
- Record only the facts: include only a factual description of the event on the reporting form, not opinions, conclusions, accusations, or admissions.
- Share the report within the system only: the report should only be distributed through a peer-review process or formal reporting program and with participants in the medication use process.
- Maintain confidentiality: forms should guarantee confidentiality and no name of the persons involved in the incident should appear in data kept after the investigation.

Where to Report Medication Incidents

Incidents should be reported through an internal reporting systems in addition to reporting to national programs. In the United States, the ISMP and the U.S. Pharmacopeia Medication Errors Reporting Program (USP MERP) are the most frequently used voluntary reporting programs.[12] Data are gathered by the ISMP and USP and analyzed by the ISMP.[9] Recommendations are made regarding prevention and contributory factors are considered and where possible addressed. For example, a manufacturer may be contacted regarding a labeling issue that is identified as contributing to errors. Information and preventive strategies are also shared with the U.S. Food and Drug Administration's MedWatch program.[9] ISMP members are informed about important issues identified from reports and analysis through regular publication in *Medication Safety Alert* on the ISMP Web site and by various special alerts.

The U.S. Food and Drug Administration also accepts reports from consumers and health professionals about products regulated by the FDA through MedWatch, its safety information and adverse event reporting program.[12] A summary of these and other programs is provided in Table 8.2.

TABLE 8.2
Medication Error Reporting Programs in United States

Reporting Agency	Contact Information	Comments
Institute for Safe Medication Practices	www.ismp.org 215-947-7797	Consumers and health professional reporting, analysis, newsletters and alerts
U.S. Food and Drug Administration– MedWatch	www.fda.gov/medwatch/ how.htm 1-800-332-1088	Consumers and health professionals reporting Adverse events, potential or actual medication product errors Action taken as needed including drug withdrawal, alerts, manufacturer notification
U.S. Pharmacopeia– MEDMARX	www.medmarx.org/ 1-800-822-8772	Hospital reporting by subscription Database used by subscribers to compare and for awareness
U.S. Pharmacopeia MERP (Medication error-reporting program)	www.usp.org/ 1-800-233-7767	Health professional reporting Statistics analyzed Further analysis by ISMP Newsletter
JCAHO Sentinel Event Hotline	www.jcaho.org 1-630-792-3700	Hospitals report and submit root-cause analysis
Patient Safety Reporting System (PSRS)	www.psrs.arc.nasa.gov/ flashsite/index.html	AHRQ (Agency for Healthcare Research and Quality) and VA partnership

Elements of Reporting Form

Most hospitals and pharmacy chains have internal reporting forms and some liability insurers provide forms. National patient safety and reporting organizations have also developed forms, some of which are available on the Internet and may be filled out online. Internal reporting forms should be compatible with national program forms so that all necessary data are collected in the same way. An example of a form is shown in Figure 8.2, adapted from forms used by other organizations.[4,9,13]

The following elements should be included in the report:

- Patient information: age, attending physician, conditions, diagnosis/symptoms.
- Date, time, location of the incident.
- Date of the report.
- Type of incident (e.g., incorrect drug, incorrect dosage).
- Facts surrounding the incident.
- Effects of the incident on the patient, immediately and up to 24 to 48 hours thereafter.
- Individuals advised of the event and date of notification.
- Name of individual completing the report.
- Names, opinions, conclusions, admissions, criticisms, or blame are *not* included.

It is not enough just to fill out a report. The key thing is how the report is used. The most important use of incident reporting is to conduct a root cause analysis to identify immediate and system causes, leading to action to prevent recurrences of similar events.

ROOT CAUSE ANALYSIS

James Reason has said that "without a detailed analysis of mishaps, incidents, near misses, and free lessons" we have no way of uncovering recurrent error traps or of knowing "where the 'edge' is until we fall over it."[1] Thus it is imperative that medication incidents be analyzed through root cause analysis.

A root cause analysis (RCA) is an investigative technique that systematically seeks to understand the underlying causes of an error by looking beyond the individuals concerned.[14,15] It includes identification of the root and contributory factors, determination of risk-reduction strategies, and development of action plans and measurement strategies to evaluate the effectiveness of the plans.[16] It results in recommendations to remove latent conditions and prevent recurrence of error. Put simply, the goal of RCA is to find out what happened, why it happened, and what to do to prevent it from happening again.[17,18]

To be effective and credible, RCA should be conducted by a multidisciplinary team and include frontline workers, not just management. It should be as impartial as possible and should include consideration of the following issues[17,18]:

- Human and other factors
- Related processes and systems

INCIDENT REPORTING FORM

Date Discovered _11/09/07_ Date/Time Occurred _10/09/07, afternoon_

Actual _X_ /Potential _____

New Rx _X_ /Refill Rx ___ Prescription Number _14569_ Patient Age _39_

Intended Drug Name/Strength _paroxetine 10 mg_

Dispensed Drug Name/Strength _paroxetine 20 mg_

NATURE OF INCIDENT:

Incorrect Drug _____	Incorrect Strength _X_	Verbal disagreement _____
Incorrect Directions _____	Incorrect Brand _____	Incorrect Dosage Form _____
Incorrect Quantity _____	Incorrect Patient _____	Outdated Medication _____

Other (Please specify) _____

DESCRIPTION OF INCIDENT:

Patient phoned pharmacy to report that she had received 20-mg tablets when the doctor had told her it would be 10 mg. Pharmacist asked patient to return to the pharmacy. Original prescription confirmed error. Correct medication was dispensed. Pharmacist apologized to patient and she accepted this.

Was Drug Received by Patient? No___/Yes _X_

   If yes, was drug ingested? No _X_ /Yes ___

   If yes, what intervention was required?_____

PATIENT OUTCOME: _Patient was concerned but accepted apology and explanation from pharmacist. She then received the proper dose._

Patient Contacted By: ____M. Rantucci____ Date and Time: _11/09/07 at 2:30 pm_

PRESCRIBER:

Name _J. Dobbs_ Phone Number: _604-551-9331_

Prescriber Contacted: No _X_ /Yes ___

   If yes, name of person contacting prescriber:_____

   Date and Time:_____

   Prescriber's comments:_____

IDENTIFIED CAUSES OF INCIDENT: _Pharmacist possibly fatigued due to working without break for 5 hours. Pharmacist misread the prescription and assumed it was the 20 mg strength out of habit as this is most frequently used. Pharmacist completed all phases of dispensing without check by technician, who was busy elsewhere._

CORRECTIVE ACTION(S) TAKEN: _Policy to ensure all prescriptions checked regardless of who fills them. Ensure pharmacist has regular breaks from dispensing to avoid loss of concentration._

INCIDENT DISCOVERED BY: pharmacist____/ pharmacy technician ____/ physician ____/ nurse ____/ patient _X_ / patient caregiver____

FIGURE 8.2 Example an incident reporting form.

TABLE 8.3
Steps in Root Cause Analysis of a Medication Error

Develop event-flow diagrams	Initial diagram: Depict the sequence of events leading up to the adverse event Intermediate diagram: Question why each event in the initial diagram occurred Final diagram: Answer questions posed
Develop causal statements	Consider potential root cause/contributing factors
Cause-and-effect diagram	Review the event diagram and clarify the problem statement Brainstorm a list of causes and choose the most important Complete the causal chain Conclude the investigation by developing root cause/contributory factor statements
List recommended actions	Stronger actions Intermediate actions Weaker actions
List outcomes	

Source: DeRosier J, Stalhandske E, et al. NCPS root cause analysis tools. U.S. Department of Veterans Affairs/National Center for Patient Safety. Available at: www.va.gov/ncps/CogAids/RCA/index.html. Accessed November 2006.

- Underlying cause-and-effect systems analyzed through a series of "why" questions
- Risks and their potential contributions
- Potential improvements in processes or systems

A framework for a RCA for a medical error has been developed by the Joint Commission on Accreditation of Healthcare Organizations (JCAHO), including worksheets that would be best suited to an institutional setting.[19] The U.S. Department of Veterans Affairs National Center for Patient Safety (NCPS) has also devised a tool for conducting a RCA.[18] It uses flow diagrams that lead an individual or team to investigate the incident through various activities summarized in Table 8.3.[18] This tool could be adapted for use in a community pharmacy, as described below.

Develop Event-Flow Diagrams

A series of diagrams help the investigators to develop a shared understanding of what happened, avoiding differing interpretations of the event. Several flow diagrams (initial, intermediate, and final) are developed that reflect what actually occurred chronologically. The site of the event and activities there should be observed by the investigator to fully understand the process.[18]

All aspects of the medication use process should be reviewed for inclusion in the flow diagrams, identifying points in the process where a problem which contributed to the incident occurred. The medication use process includes all points starting with the decision to prescribe the drug and the writing of the prescription by the prescriber, through to dispensing, delivery, and administration to the patient and subsequent monitoring. The most likely failure points in the medication use process include the following:

- Selection of drug to prescribe and writing of prescription by prescriber
- Prescription order received (may be verbal/written/electronic)
- Interpretation and entering of order
- Dispensing process
- Distribution process
- Administration of medication to patient
- Monitoring of medication

These should be considered in carrying out the steps in the development of the final flow diagram.

The Initial Diagram

The initial diagram outlines the progression of the story of the event from start to finish of the known facts in chronological order.[18] For example, the following event was reported: An elderly man received a 30-day supply of Razadyne (galantamine) for Alzheimer's disease.[20] When he returned a month later for a refill of the medication, the pharmacist discovered that the medication should have been Rozerem (ramelteon), a sleep aid. The initial diagram would appear as shown in Figure 8.3.

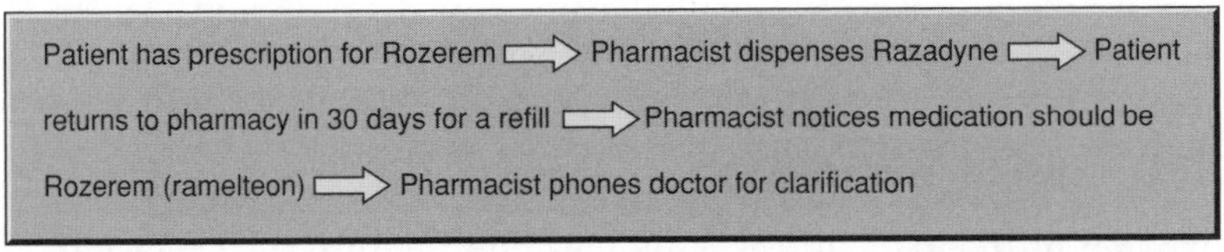

Patient has prescription for Rozerem ⟹ Pharmacist dispenses Razadyne ⟹ Patient returns to pharmacy in 30 days for a refill ⟹ Pharmacist notices medication should be Rozerem (ramelteon) ⟹ Pharmacist phones doctor for clarification

FIGURE 8.3 Initial event flow diagram for example RCA. (Source: DeRosier J, Stalhandske E, et al. NCPS root cause analysis tools. U.S. Department of Veterans Affairs/National Center for Patient Safety. Available at: www.va.gov/ncps/CogAids/RCA/index.html. Accessed November 2006.)

The Intermediate Diagram

The intermediate diagram is developed from the initial diagram by questioning why each event occurred.[18] When the "why?" questions are developed, they

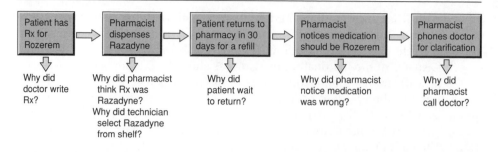

FIGURE 8.4 Intermediate event flow diagram for example RCA. (Source: DeRosier J, Stalhandske E, et al. NCPS root cause analysis tools. U.S. Department of Veterans Affairs/National Center for Patient Safety. Available at: www.va.gov/ncps/CogAids/RCA/index.html. Accessed November 2006.)

should not end in blaming an individual or group. If necessary, people involved should be interviewed and references concerning patient safety should be consulted. The U.S. Department of Veterans Affairs RCA tool provides many questions to help identify system and process issues.[18] The questions should keep delving as deep as possible. For example:

> *Initial Question:* Why was the wrong drug selected from the shelf?
> *Answer:* Because the pharmacist told the technician to select it.
> *Deeper Questions:* Why did the technician follow the pharmacist's direction? Did she also misread the drug? Did she not want to question the pharmacist's judgment?

The intermediate diagram for the example incident is shown in Figure 8.4.

Final Event Flow Diagram

The final event flow diagram answers the questions posed and also considers the relevance of these facts.[18] The final event flow diagram for the example incident is shown in Figure 8.5.

Develop Causal Statements

The next step in the RCA process involves delving into the cause and effect of the event.[18] The causes are considered by brainstorming a list of potential causes. Suggestions should not be judged, but rather all should be considered for relevance. There is no limit to the number of causes that could be suggested, but three to five is most effective. A full range of root causes should be considered, as discussed in previous chapters, including such things as communication issues, human resources, psychological issues, technology support, and the environment.[19]

When the investigator is considering possible causes, the five rules of causation used in the VA RCA tool should be observed as described and shown in the examples below[21]:

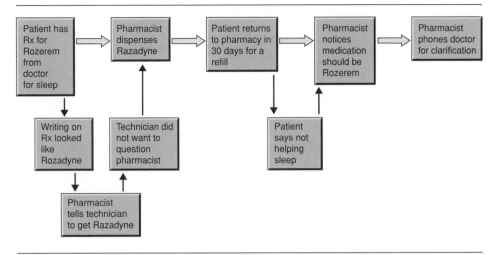

FIGURE 8.5 Final event flow diagram for example RCA. (Source: DeRosier J, Stalhandske E, et al. NCPS Root cause analysis tools. U.S. Department of Veterans Affairs/National Center for Patient Safety. Available at: www.va.gov/ncps/CogAids/RCA/index.html. Accessed November 2006.)

- Rule 1: Show the cause-and-effect relationship clearly.[21]

  Wrong way: Pharmacist misread the prescription.
  Right way: The writing on the prescription was unclear. The name of the drug looked similar to that of another.

- Rule 2: Avoid using negative and vague words. Use specific and accurate words to describe what happened.[21]

  Wrong way: Technician selected the wrong drug from the shelf.
  Right way: The selection of the drug from the shelf was done by verbal direction rather than by technician conducting an independent review of the prescription, which resulted in missing the opportunity for a second check of the written order.

- Rule 3: Identify the root cause of the error rather than just human error.[21]

  Wrong way: Pharmacist did not counsel the patient.
  Right way: Pressure to complete prescriptions for several waiting people resulting in omission of patient counseling about knowledge of the medication and what to expect, so the patient and pharmacist did not notice anything wrong.

- Rule 4. Identify the root cause of procedure violations.[21]

  Wrong way: The technician did not independently check the order.
  Right way: The prescription was very unclear and so the pharmacist interpreted it and verbally directed the technician to select the drug.

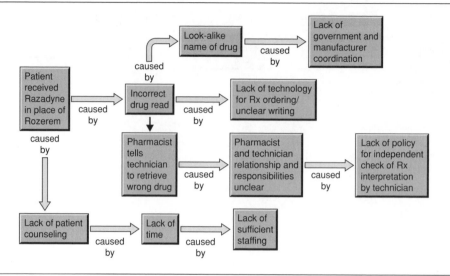

FIGURE 8.6 Cause-and-effect diagram for example RCA. (Source: DeRosier J, Stalhandske E, et al. NCPS root cause analysis tools. U.S. Department of Veterans Affairs/National Center for Patient Safety. Available at: www.va.gov/ncps/CogAids/RCA/index.html. Accessed November 2006.)

- Rule 5: A failure to act is a cause only when there was a policy or rule to act.

    Wrong way: Technician neglected to independently check the order.
    Right way: There was no preestablished policy or procedure to ensure that the technician reviewed the prescription order independent of the pharmacist as a double check of correct interpretation of a written order.

The final list of root causes should include all relevant causes, so that if any of the causes was omitted, the event would probably not have occurred.[18] The cause-and-effect diagram for the example can thus be constructed as shown in Figure 8.6.

List Actions

The investigator can then identify actions that can be implemented to prevent a similar type of incident from occurring.[18] The actions should meet the following criteria[18]:

- The root causes of the error are addressed
- Well described and specific
- Possible to implement and understand
- Agreed upon by those involved in the system and system managers

Actions may range from stronger to intermediate to weaker actions based on their ability to be most useful and most likely to be successful in bringing about change.[18]

Stronger Actions

In the case of the example RCA, stronger actions might include:

- Requesting that the manufacturer change the name of the drug or modify labeling to distinguish the two drugs.
- Instituting failure mode effect analysis (FMEA) for new products to check if they have names similar to other existing drugs (to be discussed further in Chapter 9) so that preventive action can be taken before an error occurs

Intermediate Actions

In the case of the example RCA, intermediate actions might include:

- Implement electronic prescribing
- Change storage practices
- Increase staff or improve efficiency to ensure time for patient counseling

Weaker Actions

In the case of the example RCA, weaker actions might include:

- Publicizing the incident in a report or newsletter.
- Instituting a policy to ensure independent checks of prescription orders by technician, counseling of new prescription by the pharmacist, and documenting them by an initial on the prescription
- Encouraging staff to report other situations where drug names may be similar
- Clarifying relationships and roles of pharmacist and technician

Unfortunately, not all of the strategies can always be implemented by the people conducting the analysis, nor can they always happen within a desired time frame. Appropriate reporting of incidents may make it more likely that system changes will be put into place when evidence of multiple incidents is noted as a result of an identified system problem.

Outcomes

When the RCA report has been distributed, there needs to be an outcome measure that it was effective and worthwhile.[18] This can be done by including in the report a list of measures that can be used to confirm that desired changes have been accomplished. The importance of this is also that pharmacy staff members see the value of the RCA process and of incident reporting and are encouraged to continue to do it. Outcome measures should not determine only that an action was taken but also that it made a difference.[18] If appropriate, it should be quantifiable, such as a percentage rather than just "improvement has occurred." The measure should specify how it should be carried out and in what time frame (e.g., by a random sample of 10 prescriptions per day checked for correct drug dispensed). The measures should, however, be realistic in terms of what can reasonably be accomplished.

Some outcomes that could be suggested for the example RCA would be as follows:

- FMEA is conducted on 100% of new products in the pharmacy in the next 6 months
- 90% of a random sample of 10 prescriptions per day have technician initial to show independent check was made
- 90% of a random sample of 10 prescriptions per day have pharmacist initial to document that patients receiving new prescriptions were counseled or arrangements made to counsel by pharmacist

COMMUNICATION OF A MEDICATION INCIDENT/DISCLOSURE

Dealing with a medication incident is a difficult situation that requires the use of appropriate communication skills and techniques. Looking at the protocol for handling a medication incident described at the beginning of this chapter, it is evident that communication is a critical part of the process right from the beginning, when the patient reports the incident or the pharmacist contacts the patient to inform him or her of the incident; communicating with the physician if necessary; discussing with staff members; and finally talking with the patient for follow-up.

Communication Difficulties in Dealing with a Medication Incident

The following situation describes the difficulties of dealing with a medication incident in a community pharmacy.

A middle aged female patient comes into the pharmacy and hands the pharmacist a partly used bottle of antibiotic liquid.

Patient: *(looking and sounding angry, speaking in a loud voice)* I don't know what kind of place you're running here, but you almost killed my baby!

Pharmacist: *(looking shocked and nervous)* Let me see the name of the patient and I'll look it up.

Patient: *(still fuming)* It's for my son Joseph Parry and he's allergic to antibiotics, you know.

Pharmacist: *(sounding evasive)* I'll check his profile and see if it states that on the file.

Patient: *(cutting in angrily)* I don't care what your computer says, the fact is you screwed up.

Pharmacist: *(feeling threatened and starting to get angry)* Just hold on, we just follow the doctor's orders, you know. And I see here that it doesn't say your son is allergic to penicillin.

Patient: Nobody asked me about that here. The doctor should know.

Pharmacist: *(sounding relieved)* Anyway, this order was for a cephalosporin, a different class of antibiotic that usually isn't a problem.

Patient: *(exasperated)* This is amoxicillin, not a cephalosporin or whatever. He has had a reaction to this before.

Pharmacist: *(realizing that an error was made but trying to be evasive)* Well if you didn't tell us about an allergy then we can't put that information into the computer. I usually ask when I'm dispensing antibiotics, but I guess Janet, who filled this, didn't do that.

Patient: *(still a little angry)* Sure, just pass the buck.

Pharmacist: *(sounding indignant and noticing that other patients are listening and waiting to be served)* Well, accidents happen. I'll give you the right antibiotic now if you wait until I finish with these other patients.

Patient: You'd better give me the right thing this time. And I'll be calling (the state regulatory body) to report this, you can be sure.

The pharmacist in this situation did not handle the situation as suggested in the protocol, and so it was not dealt with appropriately. He also used poor communication techniques: he became emotional, he did not empathize, he failed to gather appropriate information, he passed the buck, he did not use a private area, and he did not apologize. There will likely be a number of negative outcomes from this including loss of a customer (as well as possibly other customers who overheard), loss of patient's confidence in the health care system, and possible legal and regulatory actions.

Disclosure Communication Techniques

How things are said—the tone of voice, the words used, the attitude and approach of the pharmacist—are all key factors in creating an outcome that will be satisfying to both the patient and the pharmacist. The following are some communication techniques and suggested dialogue.[22–24]

Be Prepared

As discussed above, the pharmacist should be aware of the plan for handling medication incidents as part of employee training. All pharmacy staff members should be prepared to follow a protocol for handling a medication incident so that they will know exactly what steps to take when one occurs.

Deal with and Understand Personal Emotions

The first thing a pharmacy staff member may feel when an incident occurs is panic, particularly if the seriousness of the outcome is not yet known. They must make every effort to stay calm, making a conscious effort to breathe deeply and focus on the problem at hand without letting his or her imagination take hold with thoughts of tragic outcomes. Engaging in positive self-talk (repeating such things as "stay calm," "just take it one step at a time," "find out what happened before panicking") can help.

Choose Words Carefully

It should be recognized that words are powerful and particular care should be taken to avoid "trigger" words and questions. These are words and questions that tend to raise emotions or lead to further questions or concerns.

In speaking with anyone about a medication incident, it is recommended that the words "error" and "mistake" not be used, as they are loaded with blame and can trigger an emotional response, such as anger or fear, as well as give the impression that one individual is to blame and should be punished. Instead, the term "medication incident" or "adverse medication event" should be used, for example: "There has been a medication incident/adverse medication event."

The word "but" should be avoided because it negates what was just said (e.g., "I'm sorry about this, but I'll check into it"). The words "and" or "however" should be used in place of "but."

Questions starting with "why" should be avoided because they can make people feel defensive. Instead, use the phrase, "Is there a reason?"

The word "problem" is also best avoided because it has a negative connotation. In its place the words "issue," "question," or "situation" can be used.

Helping words and words of agreement should be used as much as possible. This can include phrases such as[24]:

- "You're right, this shouldn't have happened"
- "That may be, and. . . ."
- "It may seem that way, and. . . ."
- "I'm as concerned about this as you are."

Focus on the Patient

It is important to focus on the patient as an individual rather than the plight of individual staff members or the repercussions for the pharmacy. It should be remembered that the patient is the injured party and the staff member's personal concerns are secondary, even if his or her instinct may be for self-protection.

Be Aware of Nonverbal Language

The pharmacist should portray confidence and caring through positive body language such as:

- Stand erect with chin up
- Nod when listening to the patient
- Keep your voice low
- Take deep breaths, since the voice tends to rise in pitch when one is nervous

Empathize with the Patient

Even before asking questions and verifying that an incident has occurred, the pharmacist should empathize with the patient's feelings. Empathy is the ability to put yourself in another's shoes and to demonstrate that you understand how he or she is feeling. It shows caring and a willingness to listen.[23]

Following a medication incident, a patient is probably experiencing a variety of emotions, including fear, anger, frustration, indignation, loss of trust, inconvenience, etc. The pharmacist needs to acknowledge these feelings before beginning to ask questions.

To demonstrate empathy the pharmacist should tell the patient that he or she recognizes and understands the patient's feelings through such statements as:

- "I can see that you're very worried about this."
- "I understand why you would feel angry about this."
- "This must be frightening for you."

Deal with Anger Appropriately

If the patient expresses anger, the pharmacist should allow this to happen and not take offense. The anger should not be taken personally. The pharmacist needs to be empathetic and acknowledge the anger by saying, for example: "You have every reason to be concerned and upset about this situation, and we are too."

Reassure the Patient

The pharmacist needs to reassure the patient that the situation will be handled appropriately, that this is not a usual occurrence, and that the pharmacist is genuinely concerned. False reassurance that everything will be all right and no harm will result must not be given until it is clear that it is true. At the beginning of the encounter, the pharmacist cannot reassure the patient that everything will be all right until further questions have been answered and the situation is investigated further.

As discussed below, the pharmacist should ask questions to make sure that the patient is all right; if there is any indication that there has been a negative effect, the appropriate advice and referral should be given.

Explain the Need to Investigate

Once the patient has calmed down, the pharmacist needs to explain that a few questions must be asked so that an investigation into what happened can begin.

Avoid Leading Questions or Blaming

In investigating, the pharmacist should be careful to avoid leading questions, ensuring that the questions are not biased or attributing any blame. For example, avoid asking questions such as: "Didn't you check that it was your name on the label before you took it?"

Ask Appropriate Questions

The statement, "In order for me to help you, I need to find out . . ." should be used to introduce the various pertinent questions. These should be open questions whereby the patient cannot just answer yes or no. This allows the pharmacist to gather as much information as possible. Questioning should allow determination if an error has been made, the nature of the error, and the seriousness of the incident; that is how much of the medication was taken and what was the effect on the patient. Examples of appropriate questions include the following:

- What medication was in the package?
- What did the medication look like?
- When did you get the medication?
- Is it different from what you had last time?
- What did the doctor tell you about how to take the medication?
- How much exactly have you taken?
- How many doses have you taken?
- How are you feeling now?"

Do Not Place Blame or Make Excuses

Throughout the handling of the situation, blame must not be placed either on the patient, the physician, or another pharmacist. Excuses should also be avoided, and it is best not to make statements such as:

- "We're only human."
- "We were very busy."
- "These things happen."
- "It's no big deal."
- "It's not really dangerous."

Explain What Will Be Done

Once the seriousness of the situation has been determined, the pharmacist should tell the patient whether the doctor will be informed and what will be done next. The patient should be told that an investigation will be conducted to determine the causes of the discrepancy and actions will be taken to prevent recurrence. The patient should be assured that this is being taken very seriously and they will be informed of the outcome of the investigation.

Apologize Sincerely and Thank the Patient

Whatever the outcome or the attitude of the patient, the pharmacist should always end the discussions by apologizing sincerely and thanking the patient for his or her understanding and patience, for bringing this issue to light, and for continuing to patronize the pharmacy.

Follow-up

When the investigation is complete, the pharmacist should follow-up with the patient to provide an explanation and further apology and thanks. A formal letter of apology from the pharmacist and pharmacy manager would also be an appropriate gesture.

Dealing with a Medication Incident Appropriately

The following counseling situation uses the communication techniques discussed earlier in this chapter (see "Communication Difficulties in Dealing with a Medication Incident") to handle the incident in a more appropriate manner.

Patient: *(looking and sounding angry speaking in a loud voice)* I don't know what kind of place you are running here, but you almost killed my baby!

Pharmacist: *(keeping a calm and empathetic tone).* I can see that you're very upset and worried about this. Let's sit down over here so that I can look into this properly. (Takes bottle from mother and checks name as he moves into a private area with the patient.)

Patient: *(still looking and sounding annoyed)* My son is allergic to this medication.

Pharmacist: *(empathetic tone)* That must be very frightening for you, Mrs. Parry. Has Joseph taken any of the medication?

Patient: *(cutting in angrily)* Yes; he took three doses.

Pharmacist: *(calmly)* Is he showing any signs of a reaction—a rash or difficulty breathing?

Patient: *(calmer)* Well no, I think Joseph is OK.

Pharmacist: *(sounding confident)* That's good. Keep an eye out for a rash or difficulty breathing and take him to the doctor or emergency service is you see any signs.

Patient: OK.

Pharmacist: It's good that you noticed the discrepancy before he took more. I'll look at his profile and check the details of the prescription. I wasn't here when it was filled.

Patient: *(still a little angry)* Sure, just pass the buck.

Pharmacist: *(controlling his own anger and speaking in a calm voice)* It may seem like that, but I'm just trying to explain why I need to look at the computer. Again, I'm sorry if you're upset.

Patient: *(calming down and feeling sorry for insulting the pharmacist)* OK. I shouldn't have become so worked up. But he is allergic to penicillin.

Pharmacist: *(empathetic tone)* That's OK. You have had a lot to worry about. I see that we did not have a notation about the penicillin allergy, and also that a cephalosporin was prescribed. It seems that the incorrect medication was dispensed.

Patient: *(feeling vindicated)* I knew it was wrong.

Pharmacist: I apologize for this. I'll make sure you get the correct medication right away. I will call the doctor to let her know what happened and I'll follow up with the other pharmacy staff members to see how this happened.

Patient: Thank you. I think Joseph will be OK.

Pharmacist: I want to assure you that this is taken very seriously. A full investigation will be made and we'll let you know the outcome and what will be done to prevent such a thing happening again. Thank you for being so understanding.

In this scenario, the pharmacist was empathetic with the patient's anger, took her to a private area, apologized and admitted the error, and took responsibility for handling an investigation. He also ensured that the patient was safe and assured the patient that actions would be taken to make sure that such a situation would not recur, recovering the patient's confidence in the pharmacy.

Communication with the Physician

If the investigation reveals that the patient has ingested a medication that poses a high risk or has missed receiving the correct medication (which would therefore compromise his or her health, as in the case of missed diabetes or chemotherapy drugs), it becomes necessary to inform the physician.

As in the communication recommended with the patient, the best approach is to be honest and calm. The pharmacist should speak directly to the physician and never give the message to a third party. The situation should be explained as clearly as possible—the physician needs to know what the patient received, when he or she received it, how much was taken, and the effect on the patient.

It is not necessary to give explanations about why an incident happened or who was involved. If the physician asks about this, he or she should be told that it is being investigated. The physician should be assured that an investigation will be conducted and that this is not a regular occurrence. As with the patient communication, the words being used must be carefully chosen, and it is best to avoid the word "error."

STAFF ISSUES DURING A MEDICATION INCIDENT

Health professionals find involvement in a medication incident very distressing, particularly if it constitutes serious error resulting in patient harm or death. Following a medication incident, the psychological well-being of staff should be considered. It is not uncommon for individuals involved in an incident to lose self-confidence and possibly become anxious, depressed, or traumatized in the aftermath. The incident should be discussed with staff in an empathetic manner to help deal with the trauma. If necessary, psychological counseling should be available.

Although the recommendation is to move to a no-blame, no-fault system, the issue of culpability does need to be dealt with. The UK National Health Service (NHS) has developed a process to help managers deal fairly and consistently with staff in health care organizations.[11]

A combination of human and system issues is usually responsible for errors. Both issues must be identified, and those involving deliberate harm, physical or mental health, training or supervision, workload or fatigue should be identified through RCA and dealt with in an appropriate manner.

The "Incident Decision Tree" developed by the UK NHS leads through an algorithm to consider the following questions[11]:

- Was deliberate harm intended?
- Was physical or mental health a factor?

- Were protocols or safe procedures followed, and if so, are these workable, intelligent, correct, and in routine use?
- Would another individual with similar training, experience, and qualifications behave in the same way in similar circumstances, and if so, were there deficiencies in training experience or supervision?

If the answer is no to all of these inquiries, then the conclusion is that there is a system failure rather than a human one. If the answer is yes to any of these inquiries, then various types of remedial action with the staff may be indicated.[11] More likely, both human and system failures are involved.

SUMMARY

This chapter discusses the many aspects of handling a medication incident in the pharmacy. However, it is hoped that if the various issues involving awareness and prevention of medication incidents discussed in the earlier chapters of this book were addressed by all pharmacists and the health care industry, there would be little or no need to handle incidents because they would no longer occur. In order to put the information about medication incident prevention into practice, pharmacists and pharmacy-related organizations must adopt comprehensive safe medication practices. The Chapter 9 details what is involved in instituting safe medication practices in the pharmacy.

Reflective Questions

1. Imagine that you are managing a community pharmacy that does not have a plan for dealing with medication incidents. What actions would you take to put such a plan in place?
2. Imagine that you suddenly realize that you have dispensed Sonata (zaleplon) 10 mg daily in place of Soriatane 10 mg (acitretin) from a written prescription for a 62-year-old patient, Gerald Jones, earlier that day.
   a. What actions would you take?
   b. What would you say to Gerald (include exact dialogue)?
   c. Describe a root cause analysis for this incident.

REFERENCES

1. Reason J. Human error: models and management. *BMJ*. 2000;320:768–770.
2. Preparing for a damaging medication error. *ISMP Med Saf Alert*. September 24, 1997. Available at: www.ismp.org/NMewslett4rs/acutecare/articles/19970924.asp?ptr=y. Accessed November 2006.
3. Practical tips for errors and omissions prevention. *Ont Pharm*. 2002;60(1):32.
4. What to do in case of a dispensing error/incident. *Ont Pharm*. 2001;59(4):35–37.
5. Vieira-Conti C. Close-up on complaints. *Pharm Connect*. 1997;4(4):12, 13.
6. Harmful errors: How will your facility respond? *ISMP Acute Care Newsletter*. October 5, 2006. Available at: www.ismp.org/Newsletters/acutecare/articles/20061005.asp. Accessed November 2006.

7. Apologies gain momentum. *ISMP Med Saf Alert.* 2005;10(17).

8. Frequently asked questions. *ISMP Med Saf Alert.* Available at: www.ismp.org/faq.asp. Accessed June 2006.

9. ISMP Discussion paper on adverse event and error reporting in healthcare. January 24, 2000. Available at: www.ismp.org/Tools/whitepapers/concept.asp. Accessed June 2006.

10. Pump up the volume—tips for increasing error reporting. *ISMP Medi Saf Alert.* 2006; 5(10):1–2. Available at: www.ismp.org/Newsletters/ambulatory/archives/200610_1.asp. Accessed November 2006.

11. U.K. National Health Service. National Patient Safety Agency. Incident decision tree. Available at: www.npsa.nhs.uk/health/resources/incident_decision_tree?contentID= 3020. Accessed June 2006.

12. U.S. Food and Drug Administration. Strategies to reduce medication errors. FDA Consumer magazine. May–June 2003. Available at: www.fda/fdac/features/2003/ 303_meds.html. Accessed February 2006.

13. Ontario College of Pharmacists. Incident form.. In: *Pharm Connect.* 1995;2(2). Available at: www.ocpinfo.com/client/ocp/ocphome.nsf/object/Dispensing+Error+ Incident+Form/$file/Dispensing+Error+Incident+Form.pdf. Accessed July 8, 2004.

14. World Health Organization. Council of Europe. Glossary of terms related to patient and medication safety—Committee of experts on management of safety and quality in health care expert group on safe medication practices. October 2005. Available at: www.who.int/patientsafety/highlights/COE_patient_and_medication_safety_gl.pdf. Accessed July 6, 2006.

15. NHS National Patient Safety Agency. *Seven Steps to Patient Safety—The Full Reference Guide.* London: NHS NPSA; February 2004:188.

16. Hoffman C. Beard P, Greenall J, et al. Canadian Root Cause Analysis Framework. March 2006. CPSI, ISMP, Saskatchewan Health. Available at: www.patientsafetyinstitute. ca/uploadedFiles/Resources/March%202006%20RCA%20Workbook.pdf. Accessed November 2006.

17. U.S. Veterans Affairs. Center for Patient Safter. Culture change: prevention, not punishment. VA National Center for Patient Safety. Available at: www.va.gov/ncps/ vision.html/. Accessed June 2006.

18. DeRosier J, Stalhandske E, et al. NCPS root cause analysis tools. U.S. Department of Veterans Affairs/National Center for Patient Safety. Available at: www.va.gov/ncps/ CogAids/RCA/index.html. Accessed November 2006.

19. Joint Commision on Accreditation of Hospital Organizations. A framework for a root cause analysis and action plan. Available at: www.jointcommission.org/NR/ rdonlyres/C8CE68F6-85D7-4EA4-B3E0-89tFC10-75EE6/0/rcawordframework.doc/. Accessed November 2006.

20. Rozerem-Razadyne mix-ups. Safety briefs. *ISMP Med Saf Alert.* 2006;5(2):1.

21. U.S. Veterans Affairs. National Center for Patient Safety. Using the five rules of causation. Available at: www.va.gov/ncps/CogAids/Triage/index.html?i. Accessed July 2006.

22. Rantucci M. Tailoring counseling to meet individual patient needs and overcome challenges. In: *Pharmacists Talking with Patients: A Guide to Patient Counseling.* 2nd ed. Baltimore: Lippincott Williams & Wilkins; 2007:220–232.

23. Rantucci M. Human interactions and counseling skills in pharmacy. In: *Pharmacists Talking with Patients: A Guide to Patient Counseling.* 2nd ed. Baltimore: Lippincott Williams & Wilkins; 2007:139–187.

24. Quiring V. How to respond when medication errors occur. Presented at APhA 2001— 14th Annual Meeting and Exposition, San Francisco; March 2001.

Chapter 9

Instituting Safe Medication Practices in Pharmacy

Objectives

After completing this chapter, the reader will be able to:

- Describe the continuous quality improvement process for medication safety
- Describe continuous quality improvement methods and tools
- Describe and conduct quality improvement and risk analysis activities for pharmacy such as failure mode effects analysis
- Describe and conduct self-assessment activities that pharmacists and pharmacies can engage in
- Describe and conduct a patient safety plan

The previous chapters discuss many different ways to improve patient safety, including steps that can be taken to improve the medication delivery system, proactive measures that can be taken by pharmacy staff, and system changes that organizations and others can institute. Recommendations are helpful in guiding change, but individuals must put those recommendations into practice and adapt them to local circumstances that contribute to error.

Traditionally human error in organizations is considered to be caused by variability in human behavior, which must be eliminated.[1] But this variability in human behavior may actually help to prevent error since humans can compensate and adapt to changing circumstances.[1] Organizations need to recognize this and build in ways to allow humans to avoid error.[1] This chapter details what pharmacists and technicians need to do to compensate and adapt in their pharmacies by instituting safe medication practices.

CONTINUOUS QUALITY IMPROVEMENT

To institute safe medication practices, pharmacists must engage in **continuous quality improvement (CQI)**. CQI is a management philosophy that originated in industry and refers to management and staff working to continuously improve work processes that achieve better outcomes.[2] This is also referred to as **quality**

assurance.[3] In relation to medication use, this is a set of actions that aims to identify and document where medication errors are occurring and analyzes what is happening.[3] This understanding is then discussed with others and strategies are developed and put into place to prevent problems from recurring.[3] In California, a regulation requires all pharmacies to establish or participate in quality assurance to document and assess medication errors, to determine the cause, and to implement an appropriate response, including making changes to pharmacy policy, procedures, systems, or processes.[4]

CQI Process

To simplify understanding of the CQI process, a model was devised by Deming known as PDCA, which stands for "plan-do-check-act." This has been further developed by the Hospital Corporation of America (part of the Columbia Health Care Corporation) for use in the health-care industry and known by the acronym FOCUS-PDCA, as shown in Figure 9.1.[3] Each part of this mnemonic is discussed here in relation to medication safety in the pharmacy.

Find a Medication Use Process to Improve

The process to improve may be any part of the medication use process, as discussed in Chapter 8, such as the dispensing or distribution processes. For example, the interpretation and entering of a prescription order.

Organize a Team

The CQI team must include representatives of all members of the pharmacy staff involved in the process.[3] In a community pharmacy, this might include the pharmacy manager/owner and one or more of the pharmacists, pharmacy

Find a medication use process to improve in the pharmacy

Organize a team of pharmacy staff involved in the process

Clarify understanding of the process

Uncover/understand causes of errors in the process

Select the actions needed to reduce the problem

Plan the actions to reduce the problem

Do a pilot test to see if the actions will help

Check the results by analyzing the outcome of the actions

Act to implement and continue the improvement

FIGURE 9.1 Continuous quality improvement for medication incidents.

technicians, and clerks. In a health system institution, it might also include a representative physician, nurse, and member of the medical supply department.

Clarify Understanding of the Process

Everyone on the team needs to understand the process to be improved and the workflow involved.[3] Each individual and action that is involved needs to be identified. This can be difficult, because some things are automatic and may not be recognized as a step in the process. For example, the pharmacist may read the prescription, identify the product that is stocked (possibly under a different brand name), enter the name or the drug identification number, etc., without recognizing these as individual steps that are open to error.

Understand Causes of Errors

Factors contributing to problems in the process can be brainstormed with the team as well as gathered from other sources, such as the Institute for Safe Medication Practices (ISMP) and national or regional databases. The extent of the problem can be assumed from databases but preferably would be measured in the particular pharmacy, as discussed in Chapter 8. For example, the pharmacist may misread the handwritten patient's name, drug name, dosage, instructions, etc., on the prescription.

There are a number of tools that the team can use in order to analyze and clarify the sources of error and extent of the problem. These can include flowcharts, cause-and-effect diagrams, check sheets, etc., as discussed further in this chapter. This allows the team to visualize the process and brainstorm underlying causes. For example, the handwriting may be unclear, there may be similar drug names, the pharmacist may be unfamiliar with a particular drug name, etc. The team should keep in mind that there may well be more than one cause and contributory factor.

Select the Actions Needed to Reduce the Problem

The team then needs to propose actions to reduce the problem. The previous analysis of the process will help to identify ways to improve, standardize, and simplify procedures. Other sources, such as the ISMP or literature on other pharmacies' efforts, may also suggest actions to take. The whole team should then be involved in making decisions about what actions to take. This may also involve considering the costs in money, efficiency, time, and convenience. For example, the team may suggest that all unclearly written prescriptions be faxed back to the prescribing physician for clarification.

Plan the Actions

The team then needs to be involved in the implementation of one or more of the proposed actions. For example, it may be necessary to buy a fax machine and to ensure that physicians involved have fax machines, to train everyone in the use of the fax machine, and to develop a policy about faxing prescriptions.

Do a Pilot Test

The planned actions must be tested to see that they can fit into other pharmacy processes and can be implemented without undue stress and cost.

Check the Results

A part of the CQI process often left out is the measurement of the effect of actions on the process and on reducing the problem. Unless this is done through continued measurement of incidents, the team will not know whether all their efforts have, in fact, improved things, and they may not be motivated to continue their work. Alternatively, ineffective actions may be continued.

Act to Implement

Once it is clear that the planned actions can be implemented and will represent an improvement in safety, they can become a permanent part of the pharmacy practice. The process should continue to be monitored, as further improvements may become apparent or other developments may make the improvements ineffective. For example if local physicians adopt computerized prescriptions, the interpretation of written prescriptions will become unnecessary.

CQI Tools

It is helpful to use various tools to help the CQI team understand the process to be improved. Flowcharts, diagrams and check sheets are some of the tools that can be used.[3] Flowcharts or diagrams can help people to visualize steps in a process and show where decisions are made; they can also indicate where errors are likely to occur and point to factors that may affect the process.[3] An example of a flowchart is shown in Figure 9.2.

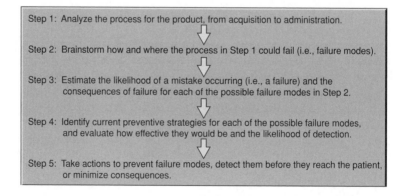

FIGURE 9.2 Failure mode effect analysis in pharmacy for a new product. (Source: Failure mode and effects analysis can help guide error prevention efforts. ISMP Med Saf Alert, October 17, 2001. Available at: http://www.ismp.org/MSAarticles/failuremode.html [accessed July 7, 2004].)

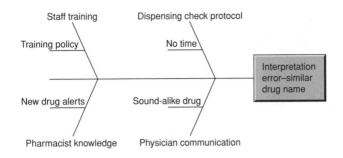

FIGURE 9.3 Example of fishbone diagram for Rx interpretation error. (Source: Shahkarami M. The quest for quality: a basic review. Preventing Medication Errors. *Quality Assurance Health Notes.* 2002;1(6):31−35. Available at: http://pharmacy.ucsf.edu/ce/qa/qa.pdf [accessed September 2006].)

A cause-and-effect diagram, also known as Ishikawa or fishbone diagram because it looks like the skeleton of a fish, can be used to visualize the root causes of problems.[3] For example when analyzing a potential error in reading a prescription whereby a similar named drug is read in place of the prescribed drug, the dispensing error would be the head of the fish, and a line representing the backbone of the fish would have lines leading from it representing various contributory factors that may lead up to an error. Each of these may have branches (bones) leading off of them as root causes of those contributory factors (see Fig. 9.3).

A check sheet is another useful tool for CQI that can be devised to record data used in the analysis of the problem. For example a self-monitoring sheet has been devised by Grasha for pharmacists and pharmacy assistants to use to keep track of their own errors and near misses, as described by Grasha.[5] An example of such a form is shown in Figure 9.4.

Methods Used in CQI

A number of different methods can be used to clarify and to take action to make changes involving different aspects of quality improvement.

Root cause analysis, as discussed in Chapter 8, is used to identify contributory factors in systems and processes following a specific event. Various risk-analysis methods, such as **failure mode effects analysis (FMEA),** and self-assessments are used to identify potential causes of incidents and where preventive actions need to be taken. A variety of other methods—such as safety briefings, safety huddles, safety climate surveys, and trigger tools—can be used for specific purposes in quality improvement. These are discussed in further detail in the following sections.

FAILURE MODE EFFECTS ANALYSIS

Failure Mode Effects Analysis (FMEA) is based on a concept from engineering literature in the early 1960s. It was originally used in the military and the airline and aerospace industries to analyze risk in mechanical systems.[6] It is a

---

Self-Monitoring Form for Dispensing Errors and Near Misses

Day:_____Time period monitored:_____

Number of staff on shift: pharmacists:____; assistants:____; clerks:____

Number of Rx you helped to fill during this time_____

Place a checkmark   beside each of the following each time near miss occurred:

Corrected Rx information when copying from telephone call or FAX:

Corrected information entered into computer:

Corrected product selected:

Corrected tablet/capsule/liquid count/measurement:

Corrected Rx label:

Corrected Rx during normal dispensing checks:

Corrected Rx as a result of counseling patient or answering patient questions:

Corrected Rx after it was placed in pickup area:

Learned of error after patient left pharmacy but prior to taking medication:

Learned of error after medication was taken:

Total ticks each hour of shift: _____Total ticks in whole shift:____

If total exceeds 6/hour, then take a break or switch to a nondispensing task!!!

FIGURE 9.4 Self-monitoring form. (Adapted with permission from Grasha A. Tools for the reflective practitioner: using self-monitoring, personal feedback and goal setting to reduce error. Preventing medication errors. *Quality Assurance Health Notes.* 2002:1(6):19–24. Available at: http://pharmacy.ucsf.edu/ce/qa/qa.pdf [accessed September 2006].)

method of assessing the risk of an error occurring by identifying problems involving products or processes.[7] Unlike root cause analysis, which is performed reactively after an error has occurred, FMEA is proactive. It involves the systematic analysis of possible problems and factors associated with them before errors occur.[7] It uses inductive logic to identify individual elements or operations in a system that makes it vulnerable to failure.[6] It starts with identifying possible ways a system could fail, the causes or contributory factors, likelihood of failure, possible consequences, and their severity and chance of detection.[6]

The FMEA process has been further developed by the U.S. Veteran's Administration National Center for Patient Safety (NCPS) for use in health care (HFMEA).[8]

FMEA should be conducted for all new products and new services to be used within a pharmacy in order to determine potential failure points and what their effects would be—before anything happens. All health-care organizations in the United States are required by the Joint Commission on Accreditation of Healthcare Organizations (JCAHO) to use methods such as this to identify potential risk points or failure modes.[3]

Conducting FMEA in a Pharmacy

In the pharmacy, a series of steps can be taken by pharmacists to analyze new products or services—for example, a new drug. This is summarized in Figure 9.2.[6,9] These steps should be undertaken by a multidisciplinary group of the people working in the area, such as pharmacists and pharmacy technicians, clerks, managers, and others outside the department or organization who would be knowledgeable or somehow involved with the product or process.

Step 1: Analyze the Process

The process involved should be analyzed from acquisition through administration.

For a new drug, ask:

- How would it be ordered and by whom?
- Who would prescribe it and for what type of patient?
- Where would it be stored?
- Who would prepare it?
- Who would dispense it to the patient or caregiver?
- Who would administer it?

Step 2: Brainstorm How and Where the Process Could Fail

The group should consider each of the processes in step 1 and brainstorm how they might fail—i.e., identify failure modes.

For a new drug ask:

- Is the packaging or the name similar to another product?
- Is it stored with other similar products?
- Does the label provide the strength or concentration clearly?
- Is the dosing and instructions clear?
- What mistakes could happen during transcribing prescriptions, inputting prescriptions, and labeling?

Step 3: Estimate the Likelihood of a Failure and Consequences

For each of the possible failure modes in step 2, estimate how likely it is that a mistake would occur (i.e., a failure) and the consequences for each failure.

The likelihood of failure could be given a rating of chance: remote = 1:10,000; low = 1:5,000; moderate = 1:200; high = 1:100 or higher.[6] The consequences could be rated in severity from 1 to 10, with 10 being very severe.[6]

For a new drug ask:

- What is the chance that the drug name or label would be confused with a different drug?
- Is this a high-risk drug?

- Is this drug used for critical illness, where effectiveness is critical?
- What would happen if the drug were confused with another, similar drug?

Step 4: Identify and Evaluate Current Preventive Strategies

Consider what processes are in place now that would prevent identified potential incidents and assess how effective they would be in detecting an error.

For a new drug ask:

- Are new drugs checked for similar labels or names of drugs?
- Are shelf markers used to alert people of similar names or labels?
- Is the name of a drug selected checked against the prescription?
- Is the finished dispensed product removed from bag during counseling?
- Is drug name on dispensed product reviewed with patient during counseling?

The probability of detection can be rated on a scale of 1 to 10:1 = very high, system will always detect; 2 to 3 = high, likely to be detected before the error reaches patient; 4 to 6 = moderate; 7 to 8 = low; 10 = remote, not possible in any system.[6]

For a new drug, ask what the chance is that:

- A similar drug name would be selected from the shelf?
- It would be counted and labeled incorrectly?
- It would be undetected during checking?
- It would be undetected during counseling?

Step 5: Take Actions to Prevent, Detect, or Minimize Consequences

Based on the findings in the first four steps, actions should be identified and implemented to prevent failures or at least to detect them before they reach the patient. And if the error is not detected, actions should be planned to minimize the consequences.

For a new drug ask:

- What could be done to identify similar-sounding drugs when first stocked in the pharmacy?
- What checks can be made prior to the patient receiving the drug to make sure it is correct?
- How can the patient be notified as quickly as possible if the wrong drug is received?

A work sheet can be used for each part of the system to list the potential failure modes identified, potential effects of the failure, severity of the effect, potential causes, probability of failure, current preventive strategies, and chance of detection.[6]

Although this method is helpful in identifying and eliminating error potential, it can be difficult to assess probability of failure and detection. It also cannot necessarily detect combined effects of simultaneous failures and is not really designed to detect human failures but rather mechanical ones.[6]

SELF-ASSESSMENT

Individual pharmacists and organizations need to assess their own environments and practices in order to identify potential risks to patient safety resulting from human failure and to monitor improvement. This can be done using an individual self-assessment form for dispensing or through an organizational checklist.

Organizational Self-Assessment

As discussed in Chapters 3 and 8, in order to properly address the issue of medical error, an organization must develop a culture of safety whereby all people involved understand and take responsibility for safety while working in a non-blaming environment. The Manchester Patient Safety Framework (MaPSaF) was developed at the University of Manchester in England and is used to assist organizations and general practices monitor their progress in developing a patient safety culture.[10] It is designed to be used by a team for self-reflection and education by using a series of evaluation sheets. Each sheet evaluates one of nine aspects of a safety culture which the team assesses both for the team and the organization on a scale of A to E.

This tool provides a framework for discussion and better understanding by health-care staff in understanding the theory of patient safety culture. It also identifies areas of strength or weakness and where resources should be directed to best improve the organization's patient safety culture. Versions have been developed for use in primary care organizations and medical practices, acute care, mental health, and ambulatory settings.

Self-Monitoring Form for Dispensing Errors and Near Misses

Grasha conducted research into process errors in the pharmacy dispensary using a self-monitoring form, as shown in Figure 9.4.[5] Using a form such as this allows pharmacists and pharmacy assistants to discover how many errors they are involved in and where they are occurring. This is for their personal use only and would not be shared with others, so that no blame or embarrassment is involved. The form is designed to capture errors at the time that they occur, hopefully before they reach the patient. Analyzing errors after they have occurred, as discussed in Chapter 8, can sometimes be difficult because all the details cannot necessarily be remembered, particularly psychosocial factors and environmental, workflow factors that the pharmacist may not be fully aware were affecting them.[5] Grasha suggested that the form could be adapted to reflect various aspects that the pharmacist wanted to monitor; for example, look-alike or sound-alike product confusion, specific data-entry mistakes, environmental or workflow conditions, or errors involving insurance requirements.

In Grasha's study, the pharmacists monitored themselves for 9 hours per week over a 4-week period at different times in their shifts.[5] This could also be done at regular intervals, such as three times a week every month, and used to periodically check completed prescriptions waiting to be picked up.

Pharmacists who used the form for 2 weeks and then set a goal to maintain their performance detected 22% more process errors, whereas those who set a goal to improve increased detection of process errors by 103%.[5] Grasha attributed improvements to increased awareness of actions and being better able to detect problems.[5]

ISMP's Medication Safety Self-Assessment

The ISMP has developed a tool that pharmacists can use to review all of the factors related to patient safety discussed in previous chapters, including human elements.[11] The ISMP Medication Safety Self-Assessment (MSSA) helps to identify measures that can be taken to make important improvements in both practice sites and in the way individual pharmacists practice. The self-assessment is designed to heighten awareness of the characteristics of safe pharmacy systems, identify opportunities for improvement, and create a baseline to enhance and evaluate efforts to improve safety over time.[11] It was developed using system improvements and safeguards that the ISMP has recommended as a result of medication errors reported to the USP-ISMP Medication Errors Reporting Programs, from consultations with healthcare organizations, and from guidelines in the medical literature.[11]

This self-assessment tool was developed for use in the United States and then modified for use in Canada by ISMP-Canada and Australia.[12] There is one tool for institutional use and one for community/ambulatory pharmacies. It is intended for use with the whole pharmacy team—including owners/managers, pharmacists, pharmacy technicians, and pharmacy students—to assess a group of pharmacy sites.

The self-assessment is in the form of a questionnaire, which is divided into 10 sections corresponding to elements that have been found to most significantly influence safe medication use according to analysis by the ISMP. These elements are listed in Table 9.1.[12] For each element, there are core characteristics of a safe pharmacy system.[12] For example, the characteristics of a safe system in regard to patient information would include having patient information in a useful form that is available during prescribing and dispensing.[12] These characteristics represent the ideal and are not a minimum standard of practice. Some represent innovative practice and system enhancements that are not in widespread use but have been found to have value in reducing incidents based on expert analysis of medication incidents, scientific research, or strong evidence as determined by the ISMP.[11,12]

Questions are asked to identify to what degree each characteristic is present in the pharmacy. Ideally, the whole pharmacy team (including owners/managers, pharmacists, pharmacy technicians, and pharmacy students) works together to assess the pharmacy. They come to a consensus vote on the pharmacy's current success with implementing each characteristic on a scale of 1 to 5, ranging from "no activity to implement" to "full implementation for all patients, prescriptions, drugs, or staff."[12]

The ISMP Medication Safety Self-Assessment is available online at www.ismp.org/selfassessments/default.asp for use by arrangement with the ISMP.

TABLE 9.1

Elements in ISMP Medication Safety Self-Assessment That Influence Safe Medication Use

- Patient information
- Drug information
- Communication of drug orders and other drug information
- Drug labeling, packaging, and nomenclature
- Drug standardization, storage, and distribution
- Use of devices*/Medication delivery device acquisition, use and monitoring[†]
- Environmental factors
- Staff competency and education
- Patient education
- Quality process and risk management

*Community/ambulatory pharmacy assessment.
[†]Hospital pharmacy assessment.
Source: Greenall JUD, Lam R. An effective tool to enhance a culture of patient safety and assess the risks of medication use system. *Healthc Q.* 2005;8(special issue):53–58.

Responses are entered online and then incorporated into a database and compared with the average pharmacy, giving the pharmacist a weighted average score for his or her pharmacy. This allows the pharmacist to assess his or her own practice against a benchmark of many other pharmacies, resulting in a type of scorecard that indicates where improvement is needed.

Aggregating results of MSSA's conducted by ISMP with hospitals throughout the United States in 2000 led to the development of the Pathways for Medication Safety educational tools.[13]

OTHER METHODS FOR IMPROVING PATIENT SAFETY

A variety of other methods—such as walkarounds, communication boards, safety briefings, safety huddles, safety climate surveys, and trigger tools—can be used for specific purposes in quality improvement.

The concept of patient safety walkarounds was developed by Dr. Allan Frankel in Boston.[14] Senior leaders in the organization go at scheduled intervals to preassigned patient-care areas of the organization and have a meeting with staff to discuss patient safety issues. A walkaround process that could be applicable to a pharmacy is shown in Figure 9.5. Using such a process shows staff that patient safety is high priority for the organization. It involves all staff in patient safety and builds trust between management and frontline staff, an important aspect of safety culture.[14]

A patient medication safety communication board or book can be used for dialogue exchange between staff regarding safety issues. This can be used to

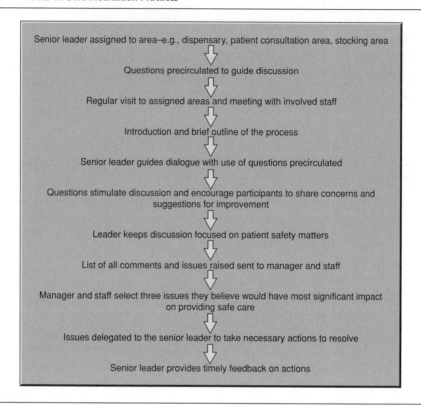

FIGURE 9.5 Safety walkaround process for pharmacy. (Source: Budrevics G, O'Neill C. Changing a culture with patient safety walkarounds. *Healthc Q.* 2005;8(special issue):21–25.

report near misses or potential risks that an individual has observed as well as noting contributory factors and recommend possible changes to avert subsequent incidents.[15] A communication board was used in a quality improvement project at the University of Alberta Hospital in Canada and was found to heighten staff members' awareness of safety issues; it empowered them to speak up and become active participants, with more reporting of near misses and possible changes.[15]

A trigger tool can also be used to improve safety in pharmacy. This is a method to detect potential adverse drug events using computer software that links patients' medical records with the hospital pharmacy system, thus helping to identify sentinel signals or triggers.[16] The triggers may be certain drugs, antidotes, abnormal laboratory values, or abrupt stop orders. This prompts a more detailed review of the chart in real time by nurses, physicians, or pharmacists who are trained to distinguish the use of drugs in response to adverse drug events from other uses, so that an intervention can be made if needed.[16] The Institute for Healthcare Improvement (IHI) has developed a Global Trigger Tool and a Paediatric ADE Patient Record Review Sheet, both of which can help to detect adverse drug events.[17]

Other tools available on the IHI website include a Safety Climate Survey 2005, which is used to assess perceptions of the safety culture of staff; it also offers safety briefings that may be used on a daily basis to share information about potential safety problems.[17]

DEVELOPING A PATIENT SAFETY PLAN

Having completed a risk analysis or CQI process for various pharmacy systems, pharmacists can then proceed to developing a **quality assurance plan,** also called a **patient safety plan.** This is a complete series of actions planned to ensure that an organization is prepared to deal with all issues involved in patient safety. By actually developing such a plan, the pharmacist can communicate clearly to all staff that safety is of primary importance and that certain actions must be taken to achieve it.

The development of a patient safety plan involves a number of components, as shown in Table 9.2.[18,19]

Create a Culture of Safety in the Pharmacy

As discussed in Chapter 3 and earlier in this chapter, a culture of safety in the pharmacy is critical to a successful patient safety plan. All individuals involved in patient care and in the administration of the pharmacy must be aware of patient safety issues and believe in their importance. Such a culture is created through the various activities discussed above in relation to CQI activities.

TABLE 9.2
Components of a Patient Safety Plan for Pharmacy

- Create a culture of safety in the pharmacy
- Lead and support pharmacy staff
- Educate staff
- Learn and practice personal and organizational preventive strategies
- Set pharmacy and personal incident reduction goals
- Conduct proactive FMEA and CQI
- Institute a plan for handling medication incidents
- Ensure that incident reports and root cause analysis are done for incidents and near misses
- Ensure that critical incidents are handled appropriately
- Implement policies, procedures, and guidelines
- Involve and communicate with patients and the public
- Evaluate

Source: Stevens P, Matlow, Laxer R. Building from the blueprint for patient safety at the Hospital for Sick Children. *Healthc Q*. 2005;8(special issue):132–139.

Pharmacy staff must be assured that the initiative to reduce medication incidents is not about laying blame. The focus in all discussions should be on the medication use system rather than on individuals within the system. There must be trust and willingness to learn from mistakes without fear of punishment. At the same time, it should be clear that it is everyone's responsibility to reduce error. Above all, staff must feel that the system is open and fair and that blame will not be involved.[20]

Lead and Support Pharmacy Staff

The management of the pharmacy must take the lead in discussing patient safety issues in a nonconfrontational, nonblaming manner. Steps to improve patient safety, as discussed in the patient safety plan, should be presented to all staff, so that everyone understands that he or she is part of the team. Staff should be supported and encouraged in identifying safety issues and in brainstorming preventive strategies.

Educate Staff

Pharmacy staff need to be educated about the incidence and causes of medication incidents, prevention, and policies to improve safety and reduce errors. If possible, partnerships can be developed with other organizations to improve preventive measures and attitudes to safety. Educational materials may be available through health professional regulatory bodies or associations. Becoming members of organizations such as the Institute for Safe Medication Practices provides tools and knowledge on a continual basis. Education must be continuous as new safety issues continually arise, requiring new preventive measures or policies to deal with them.

Learn and Practice Personal and Organizational Preventive Strategies

The preventive strategies discussed in Chapter 3 to 7 should be familiar to all staff and policies and procedures should be put in place to ensure that they are followed.

Set Goals for Pharmacy and Personal Incident Reduction

As noted earlier, personal tracking by individual pharmacists of incidents or near misses that they are involved in tends to decrease the rate of medication incidents.[5] Setting personal goals for incident reduction is even more effective.[5] Individual pharmacists and the pharmacy team as a whole can work together to set such goals, and forms should be used such as that shown in Figure 9.4, for individual tracking. Incident reports can also be collated to identify incidence rates before and after implementation of the patient safety plan.

Conduct Proactive Risk Analysis and CQI

As discussed above, there are a variety of ways to proactively identify risks in the pharmacy practice and various CQI methods that can be used. Once these are done, the results should be summarized and recommended changes described. Changes may include taking such steps as adding resources through additional staffing, technology, or software or making changes in dispensary organization or dispensing practices. A timetable should be created to ensure that these changes do take place.

This should be a continuous process through such activities as FMEA for new products and procedures.

Institute a Plan for Handling Medication Incidents

As discussed in Chapter 8, it is critical that all pharmacy team members understand and participate in appropriate handling of a medication incident. Official pharmacy forms should be created, following the suggested format in Chapter 8 or using forms provided by other organizations. This reporting process must be anonymous, and no blame must be laid during it. Reports should also be made to a national reporting program so that system issues will be recognized and addressed.

There must also be a process in place to ensure incident reports are completed, reviewed, circulated, and discussed by all those involved, including pharmacists, technicians, and managers.

Simply reporting incidents is not sufficient, so part of the plan for handling medication incidents must include a root cause analysis. As described in Chapter 8, this will identify causes of the incident and institute corrective actions to prevent future occurrences of similar incidents. All staff should be involved in this and in the implementation of recommended actions.

Handle Critical Occurrences Appropriately

As discussed in Chapter 8, all medication incidents and near misses need to be properly handled with staff and patients as well as with others, such as physicians or pharmaceutical companies, depending on the causes and outcomes of the incident. This must be a no-blame, open process so that all involved are encouraged to discuss causes and future preventive strategies. It should be viewed as a learning experience by all.

Appropriate communication skills and techniques should be used in discussions with patients and other health professionals involved in the incident.

Institute Policies, Procedures, and Guidelines to Promote Patient Safety

Policies should be put in place to make patient safety a priority. Policies should be formulated for a no-blame safety culture, patient safety goals, FMEA on new products or systems, incident reporting, root cause analysis on all reported incidents, appropriate handling of incidents, and sharing of patient safety concerns and issues.

Procedures that avoid error as well as procedures and guidelines for operationalizing the above policies must be clearly set down and regularly reviewed and updated. Familiarity with these policies, procedures, and guidelines should be part of new employee training and ongoing staff education.

Involve and Communicate with Patients and the Public

As discussed in Chapter 3, patients should be part of medication safety efforts and preventive strategies. There are things that patients should know about patient safety and what actions they can take to improve safety. This should be done in a manner so as to not raise fear or concern but rather to demonstrate responsibility and caring by pharmacists and the pharmacy organization. A pamphlet can be used, such as that developed by the JCAHO. It uses the mnemonic "Speak UP" to describe seven ways that patients can help to prevent health care errors.[21] Pamphlets, posters, and buttons are available for download from the JCAHO website and can be reproduced with the pharmacy's name. The material is written at the grade 6 level, so most people will understand it; but it would also be helpful to translate it into other languages where appropriate for the pharmacy clientele.

Above all, patients must be given the opportunity to talk with a pharmacist about their medications and conditions, so that misunderstandings do not occur, medications are used correctly, and errors are identified before leaving the pharmacy.

Evaluate the Patient Safety Plan

When a patient safety plan is put into place, it is important to evaluate the impact of it by monitoring the incidence of errors as well as staff attitudes in relation to the plan and patient safety. This can be done by collating incident reports as well as a simple staff survey asking about knowledge, attitudes, and concerns about patient safety and the patient safety plan. Ideally this could be done before and after implementation of the plan. This ensures that the plan will be effective and allow changes to be made if needed.

BARRIERS TO PATIENT MEDICATION SAFETY

As the discussions in this book illustrate, the issues involved in safe medication practices in pharmacy are complex and multifaceted. Because of their complexity, there are many barriers to the solutions discussed here. The lack of awareness of the extent of the problem of medication incidents has been a major barrier in the past.[22] In many cases, the same incidents have occurred repeatedly, partly because the occurrence of the incidents was hidden and not shared. However, awareness must be balanced, so that raising the issue of patient safety does not unduly frighten the public from seeking care (e.g., refusing to take medication or enter a hospital for fear of injury from an adverse event) or prevent health care providers from offering care for fear of committing an error or punishment when incidents occur. In addition, measures need to be taken to improve health care products (e.g., labeling, naming) without inhibiting or unduly slowing the availability of new medications in the health market.

The tendency to blame the individual health care provider for medication incidents, rather than examine the system factors that have helped to cause the incident, has also been a barrier in the past. Laying blame discouraged the reporting and sharing of information regarding incidents and therefore the causes that involved system factors were not acknowledged and solutions were not pursued.[22]

Liability and fear of disclosure is an ongoing issue for health care providers.[22] Although no-blame reporting is being instituted, there are still legal issues that must be resolved regarding liability for individuals and organizations. Legislative amendments and the legal and regulatory environments involving privacy and professional standards must ensure that reporting always occurs and information is shared between organizations. Organizations can then collaborate during investigations and develop one set of recommendations after an incident rather than various independent activities.

Nonhospital settings pose additional barriers because of the lack of organized surveillance systems.[22]

These and other obstacles to error reduction in health care are summarized in Table 9.3.[22]

Overcoming the barriers to patient medication safety in pharmacy takes a lot of resources, both human and financial. A good start has been made with financial and policy support from all levels of government and professional health care organizations.

TABLE 9.3
Barriers to Patient Safety

- Lack of awareness of the problem
- Traditional medical culture of individual blame and responsibility
- Lack of protection for legal discovery and liability which causes errors to be concealed
- Primitive state of medical information systems making timely and efficient information collection and analysis difficult
- Inadequate allocation of resources for quality improvement and error prevention
- Inadequate knowledge about the frequency and impact of errors and evidence of effective methods to prevent error
- Lack of understanding of systems-based error reduction and perceived difficulty of adapting those approaches to health care
- Lack of organized surveillance systems in nonhospital settings

Source: Doing what counts for patient safety: federal actions to reduce medical errors and their Impact. Report of the Quality Interagency Coordination Task Force to the President, February 2000 (QuIC), p. 20. Available at: www.quic.gov/Report/toc.htm (accessed July, 2006).

To address the human element, a culture free of blame is being created and there is greater awareness that there are immediate and latent causes of incidents, so that reporting of incidents and risk management should occur more frequently.

Progress has apparently been made in the United States. In 2004, the Commonwealth Fund Quality Improvement Colloquium report, *The End of the Beginning: Patient Safety Five Years After to Err is Human*, noted that there is a culture of safety and overall increase in sensitivity to the issue of medical errors.[23] There have been regulatory changes through the JCAHO, error-reporting systems put in place, and a marked uptake in implementation of information technology. But the authors concluded that there was still much to be done and gave the U.S. health care system a poor grade of C+.[23]

SUMMARY

Pharmacists, along with other health care professionals, the public, and health-care organizations are openly acknowledging that medical and medication incidents occur. It is now recognized that patient safety is a shared responsibility. Health care providers, governments, health care organizations, and patients all have roles to play in prevention.

It is the hope of the authors and contributors of this book that pharmacists and pharmacy technicians and others involved in the medication provision process will share the responsibility for patient safety and that they will adopt the safe medication practices discussed here.

Reflective Questions

1. A pharmacy receives a shipment of a new medication. Its brand name is Fanoxin, and the generic name is fonazebam, indicated for anxiety. It is available as small yellow tablet in 25-mg strength. It is packaged in a small white bottle with a yellow label. How would you go about analyzing the risks of medication errors for this product in a community pharmacy?
2. A pharmacy manager is concerned about an increasing number of medication incidents occurring for medications prepared in weekly unit-dose packages for a senior citizens' residence. What tools and methods could he use to deal with this?
3. A pharmacy chain has developed a patient pamphlet discussing medication incidents based on the "Speak UP" format. Rather than just put this on display, the pharmacy manager decides that each patient receiving a new prescriptions should be given a pamphlet with a verbal explanation. What would you say to patients when handing out pamphlets?

REFERENCES

1. Reason J. Human error: models and management. *BMJ*. 2000;320:768–770.
2. Massoud R, Askov K, Reinke J, et al. A modern paradigm for improving health care quality. QA Monograph Series 1 (1). Bethesda, MD. Published for the U.S. Agency

for International Development (USAID) by the Quality Assurance Project. 2001. Available at: www.qaproject.org/pubs/PDFs/improhq601bk.pdf.

3. Shahkarami M. The quest for quality: a basic review. *Quality Assurance Health Notes.* 2002;1(6):31–35. Available at: http://pharmacy.ucsf.edu/ce/qa/qa.pdf (accessed September 2006).

4. California Code of Regulations Add Title 16 CCR, Division 17. Section 4125 of the Business and Professions Code. 2002. Available at: www.pharmacy.ca.gov/laws_regs/1711.pdf (accessed September 2006).

5. Grasha A. Tools for the reflective practitioner: using self-monitoring, personal feedback and goal setting to reduce error. Preventing medication errors. *Quality Assurance Health Notes.* 2002;1(6):19–24. Available at: http://pharmacy.ucsf.edu/ce/qa/qa.pdf (accessed September 2006).

6. Louie C. Building a safer system: experience of other industries. *Quality Assurance Health Notes.* 2002;1(6):13–17. Available at http://pharmacy.ucsf.edu/ce/qa/qa.pdf (accessed September 2006).

7. Committee of Experts on Management of Safety and Quality in Health Care. Expert Group on Safe Medication Practices. Glossary of Terms Related to Patient and Medication Safety. Council of Europe, World Health Organization, October 2005. Available at: www.who.int/patientsafety/highlights/COE_patient_and_medication_safety_gl.pdf (accessed July 6, 2006).

8. Esmail R, Cumnmings C, Dersch D, et al. Using healthcare failure mode and effect analysis tool to review the process of ordering and administrating potassium chloride and potassium phosphate. *Healthcare Q.* 2005;8(special issue):73–80.

9. Failure mode and effects analysis can help guide error prevention efforts. ISMP Med Saf Alert, October 17, 2001. Available at: http://www.ismp.org/MSAarticles/failuremode.html (accessed July 7, 2004).

10. Manchester Patient Safety Framework (MaPSaF). National Patient Safety Agency. Available at: http://www.npsa.nhs.uk/health/resources/mapsaf?contentId=4798 (accessed October 2006).

11. ISMP Self-Assessments. Institute for Safe Medication Practices. Available at: http://www.ismp.org/selfassessments/default.asp (accessed July 2006).

12. Greenall JUD, Lam R. An effective tool to enhance a culture of patient safety and assess the risks of medication use system. *Healthcare Q.* 2005;8(special issue):53–58.

13. Organization releases new tools for reducing medical errors. ISMP. Available at: http://www.ismp.org/Tools/pathways.asp (accessed October 2006).

14. Budrevics G, O'Neill C. Changing a culture with patient safety walkarounds. *Healthcare Q.* 2005;8(special issue):21–25.

15. Zboril-Benson L, Magee B. How quality improvement projects influence organizational culture. *Healthcare Q.* 2005;8(special issue):26–31.

16. Matlow A. Flintoft V, Orrbine E, et al. The development of the Canadian paediatric trigger tool for identifying potential adverse events. *Healthcare Q.* 2005;8(special issue): 90–93.

17. Tools. Medication Systems. Institute for Healthcare Improvement. Available at: www.ihi.org/IHI/Topics/PatientSafety/MedicationSystems/Tools/ (accessed September 2006).

18. Stevens P, Matlow, Laxer R. Building from the blueprint for patient safety at the Hospital for Sick Children. *Healthcare Q.* 2005;8(special issue):132–139.

19. Patient safety plan. OSF St Joseph Medical Center, Bloomington, 2001. Available at: www.ihi.org/NR/fdonlyres/5C4C7395-9064-4580-B7c2-F1EAD4E9DC13/587/xxFINAL PatientSafetyPlanOSF.doc/ (accessed October 2006).

20. Committee of Experts on Management of Safety and Quality in Health Care. Expert Group on Safe Medication Practices. Glossary of Terms Related to Patient and

Medication Safety. Council of Europe, World Health Organization, October, 2005. Available at: www.who.int/patientsafety/highlights/COE_patient_and_medication_safety_gl.pdf (accessed July 6, 2006).

21. About the Speak Up Program. Joint Commission on Accreditation of Healthcare Organizations. Available at: www.jointcommission.org/GeneralPublic/Speak+Up/about_speakup.htm (accessed Oct. 2006).

22. Doing what counts for patient safety: federal actions to reduce medical errors and their impact. Report of the Quality Interagency Coordination Task Force to the President, February 2000 (QuIC), p. 20. Available at: www.quic.gov/Report/toc.htm (accessed July 2006).

23. Wachter R. The end of the beginning: Patient safety five years after "To Err Is Human." Health Affairs Web Exclusive. 2004; November 30:W4-534-W4-545. Available at: www.cmwf.org/publications/publications_show.htm?doc_id=250749 (accessed September 2006).

Appendix A

• •

Organizations Involved in Patient Safety

Organization	Example Activities
American Pharmaceutical Association* (APhA) www.aphanet.org	Books, products, continuing pharmacist education Recommendations for patients (e.g., "Avoiding Medication Error")
American Society of Health-System Pharmacists* (ASHP) www.ashp.org	Resources such as a patient safety Web site "Medication Use System Strategy": systematic approach for health care organizations to design, implement and maintain safe medication use system "Pathways for Medication Safety": set of tools to reduce medication errors in institutions
Institute for Safe Medication Practices* (ISMP) www.ismp.org/	Products and services *Medication Safety Alert*: online newsletters for institution and community pharmacy to report and discuss medication incidents Self-assessment tool for hospital and community pharmacies
Joint Commission on Accreditation of Healthcare Organizations (JCAHO) www.jointcommission.org/	Voluntary medical error reporting Sentinel event alerts for medical incidents including medication-related events Analysis of causes and suggestions for prevention Yearly national patient safety goals Patient safety standards incorporated in hospital accreditation process
National Coordinating Council for Medication Error Reporting and Prevention (NCC MERP)* www.nccmerp.org	Independent body comprising 22 national organizations including American Health Care Association, health professional associations, Departments of Defense and Veterans Affairs, FDA, pharmaceutical manufacturers, health care education organizations, JCCHCO, ISMP, NPSF, USP Taxonomy of medication errors, *Index for Categorizing Medication Errors Algorithm Standardized Definitions* Recommendations to prevent various types of errors, e.g. prescribing, labeling, dispensing, administering

(continued)

(continued)

U.S. Food and Drug Administration (FDA): • MedWatch www.fda.gov/medwaTCH/ index.html • Center for Drug Evaluation and Research (CDER) www.fda.gov/cder	Monitors medication error reports forwarded from USP and ISMP MedWatch receives reports of adverse drug events including errors Publishes "FDA Safety Pages" in pharmacy journal *Drug Topics* Broadcasts televised series *FDA Patient Safety News*
U.S. Veterans Affairs National Center for Patient Safety www.patientsafety.gov	Makes patient safety efforts and develops and nurtures a culture of safety throughout the Veterans Health Administration (VHA). Papers and publications including newsletter *TIPS* (topics in patient safety), patient safety handbook Failure Modes Effects Analysis Assessment guidelines Mandatory error reporting by VA hospitals
Leapfrog Group www.leapfroggroup.org/	U.S. coalition representing Fortune 100 companies who are large health care purchasers Scores hospitals on medical safety Recommendations regarding computerization, staffing of intensive care units
Agency for Healthcare Research and Quality: Medical Errors and Patient Safety (AHRQ) www.ahrq.gov/	U.S. agency sponsors and conducts research on health care outcomes, quality, cost, use and access; task forces, conferences Operates a "National Guidelines Clearinghouse" regarding quality of health care services Documents and fact sheets, e.g., "20 Tips to Prevent Medical Errors: Patient Fact Sheet"
U.S. Pharmacopeia* www.usp.org	Data collection and analysis of medication errors through Medication Errors Reporting Program (MERP) for anonymous practitioner reporting and MEDMARX for hospital reporting Publishes Patient Safety CAPSLink Service to distribute patient safety-related news Develops guidelines
Institute for Healthcare Improvement (IHI) www.ihi.org/	A nonprofit organization leading the improvement of health care throughout the world Various patient safety resources for health professionals "100k lives Campaign" to enlist hospitals in implementing changes to reduce medical errors by creating specific goals, implementation guides, presentations, tools, etc.

Joint Commission International Center for Patient Safety www.jcipatientsafety.org	World Health Organization Collaborating Centers dedicated to patient safety as part of its World Alliance for Patient Safety Works collaboratively with ministries of health, national patient safety organizations, health care professional organizations, patients/consumer groups To focus worldwide attention on patient safety solutions, best practices, coordinate international efforts to share, develop and disseminate solutions
*Focus is on medication safety.	

Appendix B

●●●●●●●●●●●●●●●●●●●●●●●●●●●●●●●●●●●●●●

Strategies and Tools for Prevention of Specific Types of Problems

Type of Problem	Strategy or Tool	Source
Accuracy of prescription writing	Recommendations to enhance the accuracy of prescription writing	NCC MERP www.nccmerp.org/ councilRecs.html
Errors with verbal orders and prescriptions	Recommendations to reduce medication errors associated with verbal medication orders and prescriptions	NCC MERP www.nccmerp.org/ councilRecs.html
Inaccurate medication administration	Recommendations to enhance accuracy of administration of medications	NCC MERP www.nccmerp.org/ councilRecs.html
	Improve core processes for administering medications	Institute for Healthcare Improvement (IHI) www.IHI.org/ IHI/Topics/ PatientSafety/ MedicationSystems/ Changes/
Errors due to labeling and packaging of drug products and related devices	Recommendations to health care organizations/health care professionals/ regulators and standards setters to reduce errors due to labeling and packaging of drug products and related devices	NCC MERP www.nccmerp.org/ councilRecs.html
Medication ordering errors	Improve core processes for ordering medications	Institute for Healthcare Improvement (IHI) www.IHI.org/ IHI/Topics/ PatientSafety/ MedicationSystems/ Changes/

(continued)

(continued)

Dispensing errors	Improve core processes for dispensing medications	Institute for Healthcare Improvement (IHI) www.IHI.org/ IHI/Topics/Patient Safety/Medication Systems/Changes/
Adverse events with anticoagulants/insulin/ narcotics and sedatives/ chemotherapy/ intravenous medications/ electrolytes/antibiotics	Reduce adverse drug events involving anticoagulants/ insulin/narcotics and sedatives/chemotherapy/ intravenous medications/ electrolytes/antibiotics	Institute for Healthcare Improvement (IHI) www.IHI.org/IHI/ Topics/Patient Safety/Medication Systems/Changes/
Errors with patient-controlled analgesia	How to prevent errors-safety issues with patient-controlled analgesia	ISMP ISMP Med *Saf Alert*, *Acute Care.* 2003;8 (15).
Errors in pediatrics	Guidelines for preventing medication errors in pediatrics	Levine S, Cohen M, Blanchard N, et al. *J Pediatr Pharmacol.* 2001;6:426–442. www.ismp.org/ Newsletters/ acutecare/articles/ 20020601.asp/
Errors due to abbreviations	ISMP Error-Prone Abbreviations List	ISMP www.ismp.org/ Tools/error proneabbrevia tions.pdf
Errors due to sound-alike/look-alike drug names	ISMP Confused Drug Name List	ISMP www.ismp.org/ Tools/confused drugnames.pdf
Errors with antineoplastic agents	ASHP Guidelines on Preventing Medication Errors with Antineoplastic agents	American Society of Health-System Pharmacists www.ashp.org/best practices/MedMis/ MedMis_Gdl_ Antineo.pdf

Glossary

active failures: Errors committed by people in the system, such as slips, lapses, mistakes, or improper procedures.

administration error: A medication error that occurs during the administration stage of the medication use process when the medication is given by a nurse, the patient, or a caregiver.

adverse drug event (ADE): An injury occurring during the patient's drug therapy and resulting either from appropriate care or from unsuitable or suboptimal care. It includes both adverse drug reactions during normal use of the medicine and any harm resulting from a medication error.

adverse drug reaction (ADR): A response to a drug that is undesirable and results in increased toxicity or decreased therapeutic effect or both.

adverse event (AE): An injury that is the unintended result of medical management.

cause: A factor that contributes to an event, effect, result or outcome. A cause may immediately precede the event or it may be latent, such as an underlying factor that influences the action and contributes to the event. There is usually more than one cause to an event.

close call: An event or incident that might have resulted in an illness, injury or accident but did not because of chance or intervention just in time. Also referred to as a near miss or medication discrepancy.

common cause: See immediate cause. Also called proximate or proximal cause.

computer-based clinical decision support systems (CDSS): See decision support software.

computerized physician order entry (CPOE): Clinical computer systems that alert the user of a patient's allergy or contraindication by using information from pharmacy, laboratory, radiology, and patient monitoring systems. This allows the order to be revised if necessary before being completed.

continuous quality improvement (CQI): A management philosophy that originated in industry and refers to management and staff working to continuously improve work processes that achieve better outcomes. See also quality improvement program.

contributory factor: A factor preceding an error or outcome that is part of a cause but not the most basic cause. It may be an active failure, a reason an active failure occurred, or a latent condition that played a role in the error.

culture of safety: Behavior and shared beliefs and values of individuals and organizations aimed at minimizing patient harm from the processes of delivery of services.

decision support software: Computer software designed for use by a clinician involved in patient care that uses information to directly aid clinical decision making. Also known as computer-based clinical decision support systems (CDSS).

disclosure: An open discussion with a patient or his or her representatives about adverse events/incidents which occurred during the patient's health care that resulted in unintended harm to the patient.

dispensing error: A deviation from an interpretable written prescription or medication order or from professional guidelines or regulations that occurs during dispensing procedures.

drug misadventure: Unplanned outcomes from medication use as a result of adverse drug reactions, prescribing errors, or medication errors.

e-prescribing: An electronic prescription order that directly transmits from physicians' computers to pharmacy computers.

error: A problem in products, practice, procedures, or systems that involves the failure of an action to be completed as planned or the use of a wrong plan.

error of commission: An error that occurs directly as a result of an action taken, such as an incorrect drug, dose, or timing of dose.

error of omission: An error that occurs as a result of an action not taken; e.g., a missed administration of the medication, failure to make a timely diagnosis, or institute the appropriate therapy.

failure mode and effects analysis (FMEA): A method of assessing risk of an error occurring by identifying problems involving products or processes. It involves the systematic analysis of possible problems and factors associated with them before errors occur.

forcing function: A design feature of a process that prevents an error by making an action or behavior impossible to continue until the problem has been corrected.

high-alert drugs: Drugs that have a heightened risk of causing significant patient harm when they are used in error. Mistakes may or may not be more common with these drugs, but the outcomes of an error are more devastating to patients.

human factors: Factors that affect safety involving the relationship between humans, their environment, and the tools they use. It includes psychological and physiological factors that prevent the detection of errors or cause them to occur.

iatrogenic illness: An illness or injury in a patient that occurs as a result of a therapy, a procedure, or other factors while the patient is receiving health care treatment.

immediate cause: An act or omission immediately preceding an incident that appears to be the natural or direct cause of an error or outcome. Also referred to as proximal or proximate cause or common cause.

incident: An unintended event or circumstance that leads to a complaint, damage, or harm to a person.

lapses: Errors that occur internally to a person during a sequence of actions because of a failure of memory. They may only be apparent to the person and not result in an actual error in behavior.

latent conditions: Conditions that exist within the system as a result of the design, procedures, or management. They may include such things as fatigue, understaffing, time pressure, inexperience, or inadequate equipment in the workplace.

latent failure/cause: A cause of an error that is result of a problem in management and organizational processes in the system. Also referred to as root cause or system failure/cause.

medical error: An error in medical care involving an adverse event or near miss that could have been prevented according to current medical knowledge.

medication discrepancy: See close call. Also called close call or near miss.

medication error: An error involving inappropriate medication use or patient harm as a result of a preventable problem in the medication use process. It can be an error in prescribing, order communication, product labeling, packaging, nomenclature, compounding, dispensing, distribution, administration, education, monitoring, and use. It can occur while the medication is in the control of a health care professional, patient, or caregiver.

medication reconciliation: A process conducted at all transition or hand-off points within the health care institution to provide correct medications to the patient by creating a list of all medications a patient is taking that is as accurate as possible.

medication safety: Medication use free from accidental injury or the activities to avoid, prevent, or correct accidental injury from medication use.

mistake: A failure or lack of knowledge or judgment that occurs during the process of achieving an objective.

near miss: See close call. Also called medication discrepancy or close call.

negligence: Failure of a qualified practitioner to provide care in a standard reasonably expected of an average practitioner in care of the patient in question.

patient safety: Medical care free from accidental injuries or the activities to avoid, prevent, or correct adverse outcomes resulting from delivery of medical care.

patient safety plan: A complete series of actions planned to ensure that an organization is prepared to deal with all issues involved in patient safety. It is also referred to as a quality assurance plan.

potential error: A description of an error that has not occurred but events or circumstances have been recognized that could potentially result in an error.

preparation error: An error that occurs when a pharmacist, nurse, patient, or caregiver is preparing or compounding a medication.

prescribing error: An error made during prescribing when a medication order is written or when a medication that is needed is not ordered. It may involve a variation from standard references, recognized practices or regulations involving the drug, drug regimen, the dose, instructions of use, pharmaceutical form, route of administration, concentration, or duration of treatment.

preventable adverse drug event (pADE): An adverse drug event that occurs as a result of a medication error. It refers to any adverse drug event that would not have occurred if the patient had received ordinary standards of care.

proximal or proximate cause: See immediate cause. Also called common cause.

quality assurance: A series of actions taken to make health care better and ensure that services or products meet appropriate or predetermined performance standards.

quality assurance plan: See patient safety plan.

risk analysis: Activities undertaken to identify and understand potential problems and the chance of errors occurring in a system. See also risk management.

risk management: Administrative and clinical activities that aim to identify, reduce, and evaluate the chance of injury or loss to individuals and the organization.

root cause: The most basic reason an event has occurred later in a system. Also referred to as system cause or latent cause. See latent cause/failure.

root cause analysis: An investigation technique that systematically seeks to understand the underlying causes of an error by looking beyond the individuals concerned. It results in recommendations to remove latent conditions and prevent recurrence of error.

sentinel event: An unexpected occurrence that is a signal that an immediate investigation and response is needed. It involves an actual occurrence or the risk of occurrence of death or serious physical or psychological injury that was not previously present that requires lifestyle change or continued treatment.

slip: An error in performance of an action generally caused by loss of attention or a perceptual problem.

system: A group of items forming a unified whole which are dependent or each other or regularly interacting such as a treatment process.

system error: An error that is a result of a series of actions and factors that are part of a system, such as a treatment process, rather than the result of an individual's actions.

system cause/failure: See root cause and latent cause/failure.

unpreventable adverse drug event: An adverse drug event that results from a circumstance involving the inherent risk of drugs that cannot be prevented given the current state of knowledge. It is not the result of an error.

Index

Page numbers followed by *c* indicate case, page numbers followed by *f* indicate figures, and page numbers followed by *t* indicate tables.